Praise for **Be Fruitful**

"For some of us, the road to motherhood is strewn with seemingly insurmountable obstacles. In *Be Fruitful,* Dr. Victoria Maizes has given us a superb, well-researched guide to help transform our obstacles into health- and life-affirming opportunities."

—Julia Indichova, author of *The Fertile Female: How the Power of Longing for a Child Can Save Your Life and Change the World*

"*Be Fruitful* is the new fertility bible for women looking to optimize their health and fertility—informative, accessible, comprehensive, and easy to reference! Dr. Maizes' sage wisdom, feminine intuition, and commitment to service are a part of every chapter. This is a must read!"

—Camille Preston, PhD, PCC, author of *Rewired: How to Work Smarter, Live Better, and Be Purposefully Productive in an Overwired World*

"*Be Fruitful* is a must read for any woman currently attempting or planning for a pregnancy. Dr. Maizes is a leading advocate for women's integrative and preventative healthcare, and her book provides practical, proven strategies for improving the chances of becoming pregnant as well as enjoying a successful pregnancy. The importance of pre-pregnancy planning cannot be overstated. As a reproductive endocrinologist, I see daily how the positive influence of an integrative approach to healthcare can benefit patients. This is a book I will ask all of my patients to read."

—Carmelo Sgarlata, MD, Reproductive Science Center of San Francisco and former president of the Bay Area Reproductive Endocrinologist Society

"It's clear from the very first chapter of this power-packed guide on maximizing fertility that a hands-on clinician, brainy scientist, holistic thinker, and compassionate, thoughtful woman is offering up the very latest and best that integrative medicine has to offer. *Be Fruitful* is an eminently readable, warm, encouraging, practical book bursting with a wealth of consequential information, backed up by clinical research and epidemiology."

—Belleruth Naparstek, LISW, BCD, author of *Invisible Heroes: Survivors of Trauma and How They Heal,* and creator of the Health Journeys Guided Imagery series

"I will recommend this book to my women patients to help them maximize wellness and fertility years before they start trying to have children. This is a must-have book in my integrative medicine medical reference library."

—Roberta Lee, MD, author of *The Super Stress Solution* and Vice Chair, Department of Integrative Medicine, Continuum Center for Health and Healing, Beth Israel Medical Center

"Who knew that low-fat milk might lower your fertility, while hypnosis could boost it? I found Dr. Maizes' well-researched book to be a treasure trove of this kind of valuable, but rarely discussed, advice. *Be Fruitful* is the perfect read for anyone seeking a happy pregnancy and a healthy baby."

—Daphne Miller, MD, author of *The Jungle Effect* and *Farmacology*

"I am delighted that Dr. Maizes has written such a useful guide to maximizing fertility. Her book provides women with a myriad of practical suggestions, as well as solutions to issues that many likely discovered through charting their own cycles, and as such, it is an especially excellent companion for those who are already familiar with the Fertility Awareness Method."

—Toni Weschler, MPH, Author of *Taking Charge of Your Fertility*

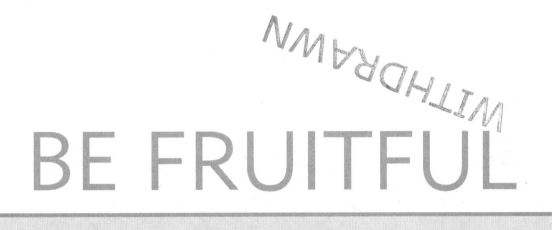

BE FRUITFUL

WITHDRAWN

The Essential Guide to Maximizing Fertility
and Giving Birth to a Healthy Child

Victoria Maizes, MD

Foreword by Andrew Weil, MD

SCRIBNER
New York   London   Toronto   Sydney   New Delhi

Scribner
A Division of Simon & Schuster, Inc.
1230 Avenue of the Americas
New York, NY 10020

First Scribner hardcover edition February 2013

SCRIBNER and design are registered trademarks of The Gale Group, Inc., used under license by Simon & Schuster, Inc., the publisher of this work.

For information about special discounts for bulk purchases, please contact Simon & Schuster Special Sales at 1-866-506-1949 or business@simonandschuster.com.

The Simon & Schuster Speakers Bureau can bring authors to your live event. For more information or to book an event, contact the Simon & Schuster Speakers Bureau at 1-866-248-3049 or visit our website at www.simonspeakers.com.

Designed by Carla Jayne Jones

Manufactured in the United States of America

10 9 8 7 6 5 4 3 2 1

Library of Congress Cataloging-in-Publication Data is available.

ISBN 978-1-4516-4547-7
ISBN 978-1-4516-4548-4 (ebook)

Disclaimer: This book is not intended to substitute for your doctor's advice. Integrative medicine recognizes that individual situations may differ and medical knowledge advances daily. Please consult your physician responsibly.

For my children, Gabrielle, Aaron, and Zoe
And for their children, and the generations that follow
May they be fruitful and multiply
And may health and happiness be their path

And for all babies everywhere, may they be healthy and happy

CONTENTS

FOREWORD BY ANDREW WEIL, MD   IX

INTRODUCTION   1
CHAPTER ONE: INTEGRATIVE MEDICINE ASSESSMENT   7
CHAPTER TWO: YOUR BODY, YOUR LIFESTYLE, AND FERTILITY   27
CHAPTER THREE: NUTRITION   51
CHAPTER FOUR: SUPPLEMENTS   81
CHAPTER FIVE: ENVIRONMENT   103
CHAPTER SIX: MIND-BODY MEDICINE   119
CHAPTER SEVEN: CONVENTIONAL MEDICINE   147
CHAPTER EIGHT: TRADITIONAL CHINESE MEDICINE   161
CHAPTER NINE: AYURVEDA   179
CHAPTER TEN: SPIRITUALITY   201
CONCLUSION: THE PAST AND THE FUTURE   221

ACKNOWLEDGMENTS   225
ADDITIONAL RESOURCES   229
ENDNOTES   239
BIBLIOGRAPHY   259
INDEX   261

FOREWORD

By Andrew Weil, MD

nfluences on human fertility are myriad. They include genetics, age, general health, nutritional and hormonal status, stress, and exposure to environmental toxins. Modern medicine is good at diagnosing the causes of infertility, treating many of them, and sometimes helping infertile couples conceive with expensive, high-tech interventions like in vitro fertilization (IVF). But modern medicine tends to ignore mind/body interactions that affect fertility and has little to say about diet and the environment; also, it is largely unaware of the usefulness of such complementary and alternative medical (CAM) approaches, such as traditional Chinese medical protocols for infertility.

With its broader perspective, integrative medicine is able to assess all of the factors that affect human fertility. Its emphasis on the whole person and on lifestyle gives it a great advantage. As well as suggesting inexpensive, low-tech interventions to increase chances of conception, a thorough integrative medical assessment can also help people decide when drugs and surgery might be indicated and how to prepare the body for them.

The author of this excellent guide is a thought leader in integrative medicine and an expert on women's health. Dr. Victoria Maizes was an established practitioner of family medicine before she trained with me at the University of Arizona. When she completed her training, I asked her to take the position of medical director and later that of executive director of the Arizona Center for Integrative Medicine, now a Center of Excellence at the university. Today she oversees the training of physicians, nurse practitioners, medical residents, and students. She also directs research projects and maintains a clinical practice. Recently, she co-edited *Integrative Women's Health,* a volume in the *Integrative Medicine Library* series for clinicians, published by Oxford University Press. I do not know anyone better qualified to advise women about maximizing fertility and achieving conception.

Academic qualifications do not convey a full picture of Victoria Maizes. She is a warm, caring doctor, a compassionate and effective healer. Because she is committed to health promotion and follows her own lifestyle recommendations with great resolve, she embodies good health and is able to inspire patients to work toward it. The advice and information she dispenses are informed by science and drawn from her own experience. She speaks with a clear and strong voice, one that is sure to resonate with readers of this book.

It has been very rewarding for me to work closely with Victoria Maizes to help bring about the much-needed transformation of medicine, medical education, and health care. Without her, the Arizona Center for Integrative Medicine would not be as successful and influential as it is today. I am honored to write a few words at the beginning of this excellent book. Rooted in the healing-oriented philosophy of integrative medicine and illuminated by the wisdom of an outstanding physician, it is a reliable and practical handbook for women who want to conceive.

INTRODUCTION

With excitement, joy, and perhaps a bit of trepidation, you're considering having a baby. This primal urge is an intrinsic part of being human. What could be more natural or straightforward? Every day, women become pregnant, sometimes unintentionally. On the other hand, many women have difficulty conceiving, which can be emotionally traumatic, exhausting, or frustrating. My opinion is that pregnancy is well worth preparing for. Whether it's ensuring that you are immune to chicken pox, taking a multivitamin with folic acid to reduce neural tube defects, or approaching your ideal weight to avoid gestational diabetes, we know that there are things you can do to prepare your body for conception and to up the odds of bearing a healthy child. Those activities, and much more, are the subject of this book.

Conception, happily, is a dream that most couples achieve. Yet we've all heard anxiety-fueling stories of frustration and heartbreak, even for people in their twenties. This anecdotal evidence has many women asking whether there's some kind of fertility crisis today. Is it now harder to get pregnant for some reason?

The answer is "maybe." The U.S. birth rate is about the same as it was in the mid-1980s (down from a high point in 1990). But the current statistics may be bolstered by the success of assisted-reproduction technologies that didn't exist in the past. Certainly there are challenges to fertility today that our mothers and grandmothers never faced: new birth control methods; unprecedented cultural pressure to be thin—and, on the flip side, epidemic obesity—both of which take a toll; high rates of hormone-disrupting stress; a fast-food diet that leads many to consume the exact opposite foods from those that bolster fertility; and environmental toxins permeating everything from our water bottles to our lip gloss to the food we eat and the air we breathe. In this book, I use the principles of integrative medicine to provide you with up-to-date information on nutrition, the mind-body connection, the vitamins you should be taking, and the environmental chemicals that you will want to avoid, with the goal of helping you prepare your body, mind, and spirit for easy conception and a healthy pregnancy.

Integrative medicine addresses the challenges to our health and fertility by synthesizing advances in medical science and the wisdom of healing traditions. In today's high-stress, chemical-laden, frequently unhealthy environment, integrative medicine is the most effective way to prepare for pregnancy, guiding you to create an oasis of health. Within these pages, you will find answers to your questions on topics ranging from the physical (what to eat, what supplements to take) to the environmental (toxins to be wary of), from the mind-body (breath work, meditation) to the spiritual (ceremony and prayer). You will also find a complete discussion of the most recent scientific findings from conventional medicine, as well as wisdom from traditional Chinese medicine and Ayurveda. This approach is proven to not only make it easier to get pregnant, but also reduce the risk of miscarriage, preterm birth, and birth defects, and, through epigenetic influences, it can alter gene expression, thereby enhancing the health of your child.

Let me offer another argument for well-informed preparation. In 2011, the *New England Journal of Medicine* reported a study of women who took antidepressant medication of the SSRI (selective serotonin reuptake inhibitor) class three months prior to conceiving or during their pregnancy. They found a two to three times higher rate of autism in children of mothers who took these medications. Now, this is preliminary research that needs further study before we advise all women planning pregnancies to stop taking antidepressants. But if you were no longer depressed, or had only mild depression to begin with, wouldn't you wish to be informed of the potential risk so that you could make your own decision about whether or not to continue the drug while you planned to conceive? At present, 50 percent of Americans are taking at least one prescription medication; the use of many of these drugs should be reexamined vis-à-vis conception. And it is not only about avoidance: two additional studies published in 2011 revealed that women who took multivitamins one to three months before becoming pregnant reduced their chances of having a child with autism or severe language delay.

I advocate for thoughtful preparation to make your body as welcoming as possible for a baby. Fertility requires health and vitality; ideally, you would not seek to create another life when your body is depleted. In this book, I focus on the integrative medicine approach, which can enhance your innate ability to conceive and bear a child. Integrative medicine is the thoughtful synthesis of conventional and alternative medicines; in keeping with this philosophy, I not only present the scientific evidence from research trials on nutrition, mind-body, and environmental factors, but also synthesize the wisdom that emerges from healing systems such as traditional Chinese medicine, Ayurveda, ceremony, rituals, and intuition. While I am a doctor trained in Western medicine, I value the experience of these traditions and the practitioners who have honed their skills through years of study and clinical practice. Within these pages, you will find the voices of acupuncturists, Ayurvedic practitioners, mind-body therapists, nutritionists, and a wide range of physicians. Integrative medicine honors working as a team, and acknowledges that no one person can know everything.

Often I am asked, "Is there an ideal age to have a baby?" Biologically, the answer is clear. Peak fertility occurs in a woman's midtwenties. For most of us, however, other factors weigh in. There are social considerations: Do I have the right partner? Is he ready? Financial constraints also influence us; having a baby and raising a child are expensive! And educational and career aspirations can be all-consuming early in adult life. In these pages, I tackle difficult realities straight on. The media has portrayed advances in reproductive technology as a panacea. We are regaled with celebrities who conceive and bear children in midlife, leaving many women to believe they can have children easily, with a bit of help from modern medicine, at age forty or even fifty. This has obscured the fact that as women age, fertility declines and miscarriage rates increase. So I ask younger women to think carefully about whether it might be best if they were to have children earlier, and I help women of all ages to maximize their fertility with the full range of integrative approaches.

In a certain respect, the challenge that we face today is an unintended consequence of the miraculous invention of the birth control pill. Introduced in 1965, it allowed women, for the first time in history, to be sexually active and to control whether or not they bore children. This freedom helped women avoid unplanned pregnancies, and drove up the average age of first childbirth from twenty-one in 1968 to twenty-five in 2002. As we swallow these pills from our teenage years on, we can lose touch with our underlying cycles, and with the fact that time is slipping by. I advocate that women become reacquainted with their cycles, as this will make it easier to conceive. It also provides warnings of potential fertility problems (polycystic ovarian syndrome, short luteal phase, and more) that are better addressed at earlier stages and younger ages when they will be easier to reverse.

Soon after the pill was introduced, women successfully fought for and won equal rights to jobs, housing, and financial and public services. We have access to unprecedented work opportunities, and building a career often overlaps with our years of maximal fertility. While social programs in Canada and Europe legislate a paid year off after childbirth with guaranteed job preservation, in the United States, we have not made this commitment to families.

The philosophy and practices presented in this book emerge from my work as executive director at the Arizona Center for Integrative Medicine. I have spent fourteen years at the center founded by my mentor, Dr. Andrew Weil, caring for patients and designing educational programs for health professionals. Our center developed the curriculum for integrative medicine and offers the most extensive range of integrative medical training programs in the world. I interviewed many of our fellowship graduates for this book, and I include their wisdom and clinical experience on these pages.

I grew up in the shadow of infertility. As a child, I wondered about my grandmother's older sister, and why she couldn't have children. My mother's younger sister, who lived just a few blocks away, struggled unsuccessfully to become pregnant. Diagnostic tests and interventions were talked about in hushed whispers; a cloud hung over the topic. As an adult, when I queried my aunt, she described herself as being "just too late." When she was forty, IVF was brought into widespread practice—but at that time, she was considered too old. Observing her sadness over not being able to have a child inspired me to focus on a career in women's health.

For more than twenty-five years, I have had the honor and privilege of working with women on health issues that matter to them. From everyday maladies to their struggles with breast cancer, transition through menopause, and desire to become pregnant, I have walked the path with them as physician and partner. I have been deeply touched by the longing to have a child, and the incredible joy that pregnancy and birth bring.

As an integrative physician, I am passionate about health and wellness. My days (and sometimes my nights) are devoted to preventing disease, maintaining health, and restoring good health in those who have become ill. I fervently believe that the greatest opportunity we have to impact health is when helping a couple prepare for pregnancy. This is the fundamental reason I am writing this book: to help you become pregnant with greater ease and to bear the healthiest child possible.

I hope you will find the information you need in this book in order to more easily achieve a pregnancy and to birth a healthy child. I encourage you to set an intention to do all you can to make yourself a welcoming host for a new life. I am honored to serve as your advisor to help you prepare physically, emotionally, mentally, and spiritually for the exciting events to come.

CHAPTER ONE

INTEGRATIVE MEDICINE ASSESSMENT

As I mentioned, integrative medicine can be succinctly defined as the thoughtful synthesis of conventional and alternative medicines. It is commonly misunderstood by people who equate integrative medicine and alternative medicine. Actually, IM is much more complex than simply being an alternative approach to Western medicine. Since we will be elucidating its approach to enhancing fertility together, I want to take you through its full definition so that you understand its philosophy and principles.

Integrative medicine is defined as healing-oriented medicine that takes account of the whole person: body, mind, and spirit, including all aspects of lifestyle. It emphasizes the therapeutic relationship and makes use of all of the appropriate therapies, both conventional and alternative. Note that there are four parts to this definition. The first, healing-oriented, acknowledges the body's amazing array of healing mechanisms. We know this to be true; if you cut your finger, the skin mends within days; if you break a bone, as long as it is aligned, the bone will knit on its own. Similarly, our bodies rapidly eradicate most viral infections.

At times, however, our bodies need assistance in order to heal. Modern medicine facilitates healing by leveling the playing field. For instance, if you have a bacterial infection, antibiotics reduce the amount of bacteria, making it easier for your immune system to fight what remains. The medicine doesn't cure you per se; instead, it lessens the bacterial load and your body does the rest.

The integrative medicine approach seeks to tap into the body's natural ability to heal, and represents a philosophical shift from the paradigm of conventional medicine, which often sees the body as a machine; if a part is broken, fix it. Too often, people think of their bodies in terms of multiple replaceable parts, as opposed to dynamic healing systems. As an integrative physician, I search for the impediments to healing, and then ask myself what I can do to remove them. Consider a hanging scale: one can restore balance by adding weight to one side or by removing it from the other. One can investigate even further to see whether the ground on which the scale stands is even. Integrative medicine values all these approaches. The wisdom lies in discerning which best supports healing.

The second part of the definition reflects a commitment to care for a whole person, not merely their physical body. Asking questions about my patient's emotional, mental, social, and spiritual life reveals the essence of an individual. A uterus, an ovary, the testes, or the endocrine system is simply too narrow a lens. In addition, I pay a lot of attention to my patients' nutritional choices, stress-management practices, and level of physical activity.

Integrative doctors acknowledge that there are two experts in the room. The physician is an expert by virtue of training and clinical experience; the patient, by virtue of her lived experience, her knowledge of her own body, her sense of intuition, and her personal beliefs and preferences. I often ask my patients, "Do you have a sense of what it might take for you to heal, or is there anything you feel you must do?" Some tell me how sensitive they are to medicines. Many women with fibromyalgia can barely tolerate even very low doses of medication; others with chronic pain may need larger doses. You, of course, know this about yourself; you know your own history of what has worked for you in the past, or what it takes to be successful in making lifestyle changes. Through engaged conversation, doctors honor that expertise, treating you as a partner in the healing process.

Our therapeutic partnership manifests in our shared interest in the outcome.

This book focuses on enhancing fertility and carrying the healthiest possible child. As a doctor, I become part of my patients' support systems for healthier lifestyles, cheering them on, acknowledging progress, and encouraging them to continue. When there are multiple options, we discuss them and decide together which to explore. Sometimes I have a strong opinion; at other times I ask where a patient would like to begin, or what her intuition is telling her. Sometimes I am asked for advice; at other times patients feel strongly there is something in particular they must do first.

I take my patients' preferences strongly into account. What gives life meaning is unique to each individual. One patient of mine had terrible arthritis. He was only able to walk with a cane around his apartment, sit in his armchair, and read; but since reading was his passion, he decided to forgo the recommended hip replacement. Another patient with arthritis had been an avid golfer; she overcame her fears of surgery and had her hip replaced in order to resume her beloved sport.

A sad counterexample occurred when a colleague of mine underwent a hysterectomy for heavy menstrual bleeding, while still a young woman. Sadly, her doctors never discussed her dreams and visions for her life with her; her future fertility was ignored, and for years she mourned the lost opportunity to have a child of her own.

Creating a safe space, where a patient can discuss her fears of pregnancy, motherhood, or labor pain, is one of my goals. Occasionally I find that women need permission to take care of themselves. More than once I have written a prescription recommending a daily walk, a weekly massage, or even an adventure.

So many people struggle with stress, telling me they don't have time for self-care. Yet it's best to get diseases of lifestyle, such as being overweight or having high blood pressure, under control before becoming pregnant. My patients and I brainstorm how to fit things in—using a lunch break to exercise or take a yoga class, or walking the mall in bad weather, for instance.

I use conventional medicine as well as alternative medicine. Pharmaceuticals and surgery are potent interventions, and I am grateful to have them in my tool kit. Still, I don't always start with conventional options. Instead, I choose the most natural, least invasive method that suits the needs of the individual. Nutrition, physical activity, and mind-body recommendations are always included in treatment plans. I may add an alternative therapy, such as Chinese medicine, energy medicine, Ayurveda, or botanicals; for others, I prescribe a medication. My goal is to help bring the body into balance by tapping into the birthright of women to conceive and bear children.

Throughout the book, you will find women's fertility stories. The vast majority are told in the women's own words and use their real names. These stories were contributed to serve as a source of hope and inspiration. I hope you will see yourself in one or more of the narratives, and find clues that may be of help to you. Dr. Julianne Garrison, a Denver physician who experienced secondary infertility, provides the first such experience and reveals the way in which an integrative medicine approach can help women in their fertility struggles.

When I think of my fertility story, I think of it more as a journey within my body and heart, than within the medical system. When I watch my beautiful, smiling baby girl who nurses voraciously, nuzzles, and turns into my cheek to give sloppy kisses, it's easy to forget we had difficulty bringing her into this world. Our difficulties began with our second rather than our first child. When we were ready to get pregnant again, I was confident that I would conceive and carry another baby with the ease of my first pregnancy. Later, following three pregnancies with three early losses, I began to worry I might not be able to have another baby.

The ache of self-doubt began in my gut after my second miscarriage when I was referred to a fertility specialist. The more minutely we looked at my medical facts, the more the theme changed from possibility to searching for areas of impossibility: blood tests, genetic tests, chromosome analyses, ultrasounds, hysterosalpingograms, hysteroscopies. With every new finding or theory, I felt more uncertain.

Eventually, my inner alarm bells sounded. I started to do my own research. An ultrasound done by the fertility expert revealed high indices of impedence in my uterine arteries (the blood wasn't flowing properly). I read that dietary changes like reducing caffeine use and increasing intake of antioxidants could increase blood flow, making my uterus more receptive for implantation. I beefed up my supplements, adding antioxidants and vitamin C. I added fish oil to improve fetal brain development and reduce the risk of preterm labor. I also found studies which suggested that women receiving fertility-directed acupuncture treatments have pregnancy rates that are higher than women who receive only conventional treatment, and some research that showed improved blood flow through the uterine arteries following acupuncture treatments. I began fertility-directed acupuncture.

Even with the aid of supplements and acupuncture, I had another miscarriage. My spirits and emotions rose and fell in synchrony with my HCG levels. As I became more anxious, I turned to yoga and gentle movement to let go and slow down. I scheduled ten minutes of intentful, cleansing breath before my first patient every day, at lunch, and after my last patient visit—before heading home to my family and busy home life. I initiated self-hypnotherapy, often repeating reassuring and positive messages to myself and to my body. Yoga, breath-work, meditation, and self-hypnosis became my link to sanity.

Ultimately, I made the decision not to proceed with more invasive fertility treatments, and instead turned to an obstetrician colleague and now friend, Roy Bergstrom, MD, who listened to me and escorted me to a successful pregnancy. With his guidance, I used conventional medications (progesterone and Clomid) in conjunction with antioxidants, imagery, self-hypnosis, breathing, and acupuncture. The ending of my fertility story is a "happily ever after" ending, but the difficulty of the endeavor will always be a part of me. Often, in the folds of many small moments, I feel gratitude. Gratitude for my baby girl, for her big brother, and for their father! Gratitude for the doctors and conventional medications in conjunction with antioxidants, imagery, self-hypnosis, breathing, and acupuncture that made it possible for me to have my daughter. And gratitude for my body, which hosted, nurtured, and accommodated

11

two growing beings for forty long weeks each and, most importantly, never forgot its innate fertility.

The Eight Principles of Integrative Medicine

1. The patient and practitioner are partners in the healing process.
2. Take into consideration all factors that influence health, wellness, and disease.
3. Use conventional and alternative methods appropriately to facilitate the body's innate healing response.
4. Use natural and less invasive interventions whenever possible.
5. Neither reject conventional medicine nor accept alternative medicine uncritically.
6. Good medicine is based in good science.
7. Health promotion and prevention go along with treatment.
8. Physicians should walk their talk.

I'll discuss these eight principles briefly here. The first is that the patient and practitioner are partners in the healing process, and that we recognize and honor the expertise of each. Individuals' goals can vary widely. One person may come to me and say, "I really want to work on weight loss"; for another, weight is off-limits, but managing stress is open to discussion. I honor my patients' decisions and preferences about their lives and bodies.

The second principle is that all factors that influence health, wellness, and disease are taken into consideration. By my taking an extensive history, and listening to my patient's full story, a healing path often emerges. For instance, I have been struck by the frequency with which a careful dietary history has detected food intolerances that were the subtle culprits behind disease. Time and again, a trial of removing dairy for three weeks has led to resolution of sinus symptoms, heartburn, and bloating; other common food triggers are wheat, eggs, soy, and citrus. Inadequate sleep can be the root cause for symptoms as broad as irritability, joint pain, body aches, weight gain, and depression. A freshly painted office may explain the new onset of headaches, nausea, and fatigue.

The third principle calls for appropriate use of conventional and alternative methods to facilitate the body's innate healing response. Many strategies can be used to enhance health and well-being. In this book, you will learn about the uses of acupuncture, Ayurveda, energy practices, and ritual, as well as nutrition, supplements, and mind-body interactions. Discerning which to use, in what combination, and in what order is at the heart of the art of integrative medicine; it is influenced by the available scientific evidence; the desires, beliefs, and intuitions of the patient; and the doctor's clinical experience.

The fourth principle of integrative medicine is to use natural and less invasive interventions whenever possible. Modern medicine can be miraculous. Procedures such as IVF, egg donation, or ICSI (intracytoplasmic sperm injection, in which a single sperm is injected directly into an egg) can allow childbearing for women and men who previously could never have had children. The advances of Western medicine can often solve infertility challenges that a generation ago were insurmountable, with adoption the only option. I am deeply grateful for these advances, but they do not come without risks.

This principle of leading with the most natural and least invasive treatments may not be intuitive to all readers. After all, in the United States, we pride ourselves on having the most advanced health care system in the world. Why wouldn't we want to use the most advanced technologies first? The reasons include overdiagnosis, overtreatment, and the potential risks and side effects of treatment.

Take the example of routine fetal heart monitoring of your baby when you go to the hospital in labor. It might seem obvious that monitoring the baby's heart rate is a good thing—you can detect if the fetus is not getting enough oxygen (which leads the baby's heart rate to slow down) and intervene if necessary. Counterintuitively, a Cochrane review of 37,000 women found that it did not improve the baby's Apgar scores (a measure of wellness at birth), lower the rate of cerebral palsy, or lower the

13

number of infant deaths; there was only a tiny reduction in seizures (from 2/1000 to 1/1000). On the downside, it increased the rate of cesarean sections by 66 percent. C-sections are not benign. Besides the risk of anesthesia, they are more difficult for women to recover from than a vaginal birth; require longer hospital stays; have higher rates of infection, blood loss, and blood clots; and raise the potential for additional surgeries. Babies born by C-section have more breathing problems and lower Apgar scores than those born vaginally. There is also a concern that because these babies are not colonized by bacteria from their mothers' vaginas during the birth process, their immune systems are negatively impacted, which results in increased allergy and auto-immune diseases later in life.

There are many examples of the risks of diagnostic tests and invasive technologies, which is why IM suggests we minimize them if possible. But in some cases, the practices of conventional medicine can be critical to the health of the patient. If you have a blocked fallopian tube, for example, laparoscopic microsurgery may well be the very best first step.

Integrative medicine prefers natural and noninvasive methods in fertility treatment because of the risks associated with this (granted, amazing) technology. We begin with the least invasive, lowest-risk intervention, as demanded by the patient's situation.

The fifth principle is that integrative medicine neither rejects conventional medicine nor accepts alternative medicine uncritically. We must be discerning; there are practices in alternative medicine that I never recommend. Just as we don't always jump to IVF, we don't leap to alternative medicine, either. Working with an integrative doctor can be helpful here, so that you don't have to sort it out all on your own.

The sixth principle is that good medicine is based in good science; it is inquiry-driven and open to new paradigms. Unfortunately, many physicians still say, "There is no evidence for integrative medicine," without actually examining the scientific literature. Or they say, "Alternative medicine is dangerous," when many of the practices bear significantly lower risk than Western medicine. Women are taught to be afraid of using Chinese herbs because their reproductive endocrinologists tell them not to, or they don't use acupuncture, even though there is good evidence that it enhances fertility, because their doctors have not reviewed the journals that report on acupuncture.

As physicians, we need to be open-minded skeptics. We bear an obligation to our patients to explore the existing evidence before rejecting a practice. And sometimes a lack of evidence doesn't mean that a practice or remedy doesn't work; it could be that adequate studies just haven't been done yet. There's a difference between something that has been proven not to work and something that hasn't been adequately studied.

The seventh principle of integrative medicine places health promotion and prevention alongside treatment. This is the underlying premise of this book: do all that you can to be as healthy as possible, in order to ready yourself to have a child. By cleaning up your diet, honing your stress reduction practices and exercise habits, and adjusting your weight if you are over- or underweight, you are preparing yourself to serve as the vessel for a developing life.

Ask yourself what you can do to improve your health, so that conception will come more easily and you'll have a healthy baby. For instance, Americans eat more processed foods than we used to. These processed foods are loaded with artificial chemicals, as well as trans fats and sugar. Environmental exposures have skyrocketed; the umbilical blood of newborn babies has been shown to contain more than two hundred chemicals before they've taken a single breath. Yet we know that when children are placed on an organic diet, the amount of chemicals found in their urine is reduced. In Chapter 5, "Environment," I will show you many ways to lessen exposure to environmental chemicals when preparing to conceive.

The last principle is that practitioners of integrative medicine should exemplify its tenets. We ask physicians and nurse practitioners to walk the talk. Instead of just preaching to others, we also wrestle with these challenges in our own lives. And in so doing, we deeply commit ourselves to the same lifestyle practices we ask of our patients.

The Initial Assessment

When a couple comes to talk with me about planning for pregnancy, I frame it as a wonderful opportunity for them to self-assess, to think about their current lifestyle and what changes they might wish to make. I ask the couple to think about how having a child will change their life emotionally and spiritually. There's a saying that I heard while in India: "The world is divided into those who have seen the Taj Mahal, and those who have not yet seen it." Likewise, having a child defines you for the rest of your life. You are embarking upon a major life-changing experience from which there is no going back.

I always start the same way when I see a new patient. Our initial visit lasts ninety minutes. I greet my patient and say, "We have an hour and a half to spend together. My goal is to get a sense of who you are as a person and the things that are important to you, in addition to any medical conditions that brought you in today." By asking them to tell their story, I'm signaling that this is going to be a different experience.

Some people launch right into their histories; others ask for further guidance. I might say, "You can start anywhere you want. You can tell me where you were born and raised, about your childhood, or where you went to school. Or you can begin with your medical concern." Often the medical issue is foremost in a person's mind, so we start there, and then move on to the larger life story. Usually the patient does most of the talking in the first part of our session, and I do more talking in the second half, when I give suggestions. By getting a sense of the whole person, I can give a much broader set of recommendations.

I have never met anyone who was unhappy with this style of interviewing. People rarely have the opportunity to tell their stories in their own words, and to be witnessed and heard. Generous listening is a very important part of this experience; it gives me a sense of the very essence of a person. I can also listen for clues about what is most likely to activate healing, and the best ways to convey the recommendations. My goal is to discern the right medicine—not meaning pills, but treatment in the broadest sense of the word.

When people see me for fertility issues, I may inquire into the stories of their own births as well as their relationships with their parents, and their thoughts, questions, beliefs, or concerns about getting pregnant. People range tremendously, from feeling that this will be easy to "I've always worried that conception will be hard for me," in which case, I ask why that might be so. In taking their broad histories, I ask about their GI tract and digestion, because that may indicate food intolerances. For example, celiac disease is often underdiagnosed, and it can contribute to fertility issues. Cold hands and feet often are a sign of sympathetic nervous system overdrive; if their peripheral circulation is constricted, the blood flow to their uteruses and ovaries may be clamped down, too.

As I'm listening to my new patient, I attend not only to what changes the person will need to make, but also to what they're doing right. At the end of our meeting, I always acknowledge their successes. I think it's a terrible error for doctors to focus only on what a patient is doing wrong—as in, "You need to change your diet" or "You need to lose weight." Instead, when I finish, I sum up with something like, "You have a strong relationship with your husband and parents, and good social support through your church. It's great that you're going for a long walk twice a week. Please continue all these habits. And here are my recommendations that address your medical concerns and help fine-tune your lifestyle."

Of course, I also focus specifically on fertility, asking, if the subject hasn't been covered in the course of a patient's story, about her menstrual periods, including at what age they started, how regular they are, what the flow is like, the duration of the cycle, and whether she experiences menstrual pain. Some women don't know much about their natural cycle because they began the pill soon after they began menstruating.

In addition, I find out what type of contraception she has used, when she discontinued it, and what effect it has had on her fertility. Is she taking any medications that can get in the way of conception? For example, antihistamines that can dry out cervical mucus and make it less hospitable for sperm. Did she have surgery for blocked tubes or fibroids? Has she been diagnosed with PCOS (polycystic ovarian syndrome) or any other condition that could affect fertility? Of course I also want to know about previous pregnancies, abortions, or miscarriages.

My patients' eating habits are very important. I ask about their relationship to food (up to 20 percent of women with infertility have eating disorders). Who prepares their meals? Do they like or hate to cook? I also want to know how often they eat out, how often they have freshly cooked natural foods, what their cravings are, about any food intolerances, how often they eat sushi, what their fish intake is, whether they pay attention to mercury, how many servings of vegetables and fruit per day they eat, how much animal protein or vegetable protein they consume, and whether they are on any special diets, such as Atkins, the Zone, shakes, or Medifast. Do they binge, or do they have a sweet tooth and eat a lot of cake, candy, or pastries? (These high-glycemic index foods bump up blood sugar, which can interfere with fertility.) How much soda, alcohol, and coffee do they drink?

Patients keep a twenty-four-hour diet record before they come in to see me. They list all that they've eaten over the course of a day, and state whether it is typical or not. In addition, I ask people what they usually eat for breakfast, lunch, and dinner, so that depending on their diet, we can negotiate changes. Perhaps instead of breakfast cereal, they would be willing to have steel-cut oatmeal or scrambled eggs.

I also inquire about the vitamins, herbs, supplements, and over-the-counter and prescribed medications a patient is taking. Some people come in with two shopping bags full of pills, capsules, and tinctures; others may not be taking anything at all. I ask how attached they are to particular products. At times, people have a strong belief in something that I don't think helps but that is not dangerous; if I have a concern about the item, I'll tell them.

Some people are on too much vitamin A, which can inhibit fertility and increase the risk of hip fractures as their bodies age. Often people ingest too much vitamin B, because B is added to so many supplements. We also discuss medications they need to stop taking, such as Accutane and antihistamines. I recommend women take a prenatal multivitamin with folic acid and iron. I determine whether a patient needs omega-3 fatty acids, based on her dietary intake. Finally, I may order lab work to test for anemia, immunizations, and vitamin D deficiency.

I like to ask about my patients' activity levels. People vary from zero activity—those who hate to break a sweat—to those whose exercise habits may suppress normal ovulation. I weigh patients to check whether they are over- or underweight, measure their height, then calculate their body mass index (BMI). You can calculate your own BMI by dividing your weight in pounds by the square of your height in inches, and then multiplying this number by 703. For example, if you weigh 140 pounds and are 5 foot 7 inches (67 inches) tall, your BMI would be $140 \div (67 \times 67) \times 703 = 21.9$. The ideal BMI for conception is 20 to 24; less or more makes it harder to conceive.

And the higher the BMI, the greater the risk of gestational diabetes. A father's weight influences the weight of his prepubertal daughter, an epigenetic effect that makes obesity an important issue for men and women.

Additional medical information that I inquire about includes the patient's thyroid function, whether or not she smokes cigarettes or did in the past, and family history. Then I go over immunizations, ask about celiac disease, and discuss PCOS symptoms such as excess facial or body hair, acne, and irregular periods.

Environmental exposures to chemicals are a huge concern. More than 84,000 different chemicals have been produced in the United States and are used in workplaces, homes, and communities; we have information about the effects on reproduction of only a few thousand. At work, women and men can be exposed to lead, X-rays, solvents, and chemotherapeutic agents. Diet can expose couples to mercury, PCBs, and organophosphate residues. At home, remodeling projects for the baby's room can lead to off-gassing from new carpets, furniture, and paint; luckily more and more environmentally friendly materials are becoming available. In and around the house, consider alternative ways to get rid of bugs or pests rather than having the exterminator spray. Wise choices can also be made about cleaning products, cosmetics, perfumes, glues, air fresheners, shampoos, and body lotions.

Emotional issues are brought up as well. I ask my new patient if she has any concerns about getting pregnant. These can include worries about changes in her body, getting "fat," or a fear that she won't be able to lose weight after giving birth. I inquire about how much stress she is under, and what coping strategies she is using to deal with it. Couples often have unspoken fears about the impact of children on their relationships. At times, one partner wants a baby, but the other doesn't.

In terms of beliefs, I inquire as to whether they believe that they can get pregnant and have a healthy child. We discuss their emotional readiness; sometimes a person says that she wants to have a child but actually is uncertain or unready. There are "wrong reasons" for wanting a child, such as to fix a broken marriage or to have someone who will give unconditional love.

We also discuss spiritual practices. I want to know if my patient has a religious practice or faith tradition that is important to her. If she is religious, I may ask her whether she prays for herself; many people seem to need permission to pray for them-

19

selves. I ask where they get their strength during difficult times. Often such strength comes from a spiritual practice. Sometimes people are not using tools they already have. It can be helpful to remind a person of something that they know but aren't currently accessing.

Below you'll find the Self-Assessment Test. While I usually complete these questions with my patients, I encourage you to respond to them on your own. Look at your answers and think about them. What surprises you? What habits are you proud of? What do you look to change or transform? Often, just writing down the answers to some of these questions can be helpful to finding the path forward.

Self-Assessment Test

Menstrual Periods

At what age did you start your period?

How regular are your periods?

How long is your cycle?

What is your flow like?

Do you have pain during your period?

How do you view your period?

Contraception

What type of birth control have you used?

Have you discontinued it?

What effect, if any, has it had on your fertility?

Have your periods returned to normal?

Nutrition

Do you cook your own food?

How often do you eat out?

Are you on any kind of special diet, such as Atkins, the Zone, shakes, or Medifast?

How often do you eat freshly cooked whole foods?

Do you have any food intolerances?

How many servings of vegetables and fruit do you eat per day?

How often do you eat fish?

Are you avoiding shark, swordfish, tilefish, and king mackerel?

How often do you eat sushi?

How many servings of animal protein do you consume daily?

How many servings of vegetable protein do you consume daily?

Do you binge, or have a sweet tooth and eat a lot of cake, candy, or pastries?

How many sodas or sweetened beverages do you drink each week?

How many alcoholic beverages do you drink each week?

How much coffee do you drink per day?

Do you use iodized salt?

What do you usually eat for breakfast, lunch, and dinner?

Supplements

What vitamins, herbs, and/or supplements do you take?

Are you taking a prenatal multivitamin multimineral with folic acid, iron, and iodine?

Where do you get your advice regarding choosing supplements?

Have you been tested for vitamin D deficiency?

Conventional

What prescribed medications do you take?

What over-the-counter medications do you take?

Have you discussed the safety of these during pregnancy with your doctor or pharmacist?

Are your immunizations up to date?

Do you have celiac disease?

Do you have thyroid disease?

Do you have PCOS symptoms such as excess facial or body hair, acne, and irregular periods?

Have you had surgery for blocked tubes or fibroids?

Have you or your partner been diagnosed with any medical problems that could affect fertility?

Have you had any previous pregnancies, abortions, or miscarriages?

Lifestyle

What is your daily activity level?

How many hours per week do you exercise?

What is your height and weight?

What is your BMI?

Do you currently smoke cigarettes?

How many hours of sleep do you get each night?

Environment

Have you been exposed to lead, X-rays, solvents, or chemotherapeutic agents?

Do you avoid fish that contain mercury and PCBs?

Do you pay attention to the pesticides in your vegetables and fruits and select those with lower levels or purchase organic?

Have you bought new furniture or carpets recently?

Have you painted the house recently? Did you use no- or low-VOC paint?

Do you spray the house for bugs?

Do you use green cleaning products?

Do you have your lawn sprayed?

Do you check the ingredients in your cosmetics, lotions, and shampoos?

Do you use perfumes and/or air fresheners?

Mind-Body

> Do you have any concerns or fears about getting pregnant?
>
> Do you have fears about changes in your body, getting "fat," or a fear that you won't be able to lose the weight after giving birth?
>
> How much stress are you under?
>
> How do you manage the stress in your life?
>
> Do you do yoga, mindful walking, journaling, meditation, or other mind-body practices?
>
> Do you believe that you can get pregnant and have a healthy child?

Spirituality

> Do you have a religious practice or faith tradition that is important to you?
>
> Do you pray for yourself?
>
> Where do you get your strength during difficult times?

A patient of mine, whom I'll call Susan, had just turned thirty-four. She was newly married and wasn't quite ready to have a child because she had just taken on a demanding job. She had talked about this with her ob-gyn, who recommended that she freeze embryos because of her age. Susan asked for my advice, and we had an illuminating conversation about it. This is the art of integrative medicine, as Susan's question does not have a right or wrong answer. The decision lies in her being true to her personal beliefs.

I made a variety of recommendations for Susan. She had been on the pill for fourteen years, so the first thing I suggested was for her to go off the pill and pay attention to her cycles. I often find that women who have been on the pill for quite some time know very little about their bodies' natural cycles; I will discuss this in more depth in Chapter 2, "Your Body, Your Lifestyle, and Fertility." I advised Susan to become reacquainted with her own body. If she had abundant cervical mucus and regular periods, as well as signs of ovulation in her basal body temperature, this

23

would suggest that she was still quite fertile. On the other hand, if she went off the pill and discovered that month after month she was not ovulating at all, I would suggest a course of acupuncture.

I made some dietary recommendations as well, such as switching from skim to whole milk, and recommended reducing environmental exposures in her cosmetics, shampoo, and sunscreen by reviewing products on a cosmetics database. We discussed her taking a prenatal multivitamin with folic acid, iron, and omega-3. I also asked her to get some blood work, including a vitamin D level. Susan is a sushi lover, and we reviewed which fish have the lowest levels of mercury. She is also an athlete, having run in nine marathons in the past ten years. We discussed reducing her exercise duration and intensity as she moved toward conception.

In addition, Susan had a few friends who had done IVF, so I suggested that she get firsthand accounts from them in order to hear what it was like. This would better inform her decision about whether she would want to preserve embryos. While none of us have a crystal ball, at least this would give Susan a perspective of what the procedure might be like.

Even though she didn't want to get pregnant for another two years, Susan was delighted to learn that there were things she could do during this period to prepare herself so that when she was ready to conceive, her body would be ready, too. Susan was grateful for the discussion because the conversation she had had with her doctor went no deeper than "You're getting old; you should consider freezing embryos." Susan's general preference was to take a more natural approach to her health; another woman might have preferred the high-tech solution. Ideally, as physicians, we help our patients select treatment options that fit who they are.

As I consider treatment recommendations, I am also thinking about whether my patient needs to meet with someone else on the health care team. Does she need the advice of a nutritionist, a mind-body group experience, or the support of acupuncture? Would a visit with a hypnotherapist be of value? What resources do I want to make her aware of? In integrative medicine, we value the strengths that different systems of healing bring to the table.

Fertility treatment can become all consuming; I highly recommend to my patients that they retain the interests and hobbies that lend richness to their lives, maintain meaningful work and relationships, and nourish the fullness of life, so that their sole focus is not becoming pregnant. You often hear about people who conceived on vacation or immediately after adoption, when they finally let go. I believe that there is a lesson there about not striving so hard. A sleep-expert colleague of mine, Dr. Rubin Naiman, says, "You cannot *go* to sleep; you must *let go* into sleep." Similarly, we cannot *get* pregnant. With every advance in the world, there is still a mystery to the creation of life that eludes us. We must let go, make ourselves the most receptive vessels for life that we can be, and allow the mystery to unfold.

CHAPTER TWO

YOUR BODY, YOUR LIFESTYLE, AND FERTILITY

Melissa came to see me in my integrative medicine clinic after several years of trying to get pregnant. A paralegal, she was twenty-nine and had married her high-school sweetheart soon after they both graduated from college. Melissa related that she had always struggled a bit with her weight and did a lot of hiking to maintain it. Melissa had gone on the pill at age fifteen to regulate her periods. A few years later, she and her boyfriend became sexually intimate. It was only at age twenty-six, when they decided to become pregnant, that she went off the pill and was surprised to find her periods were still irregular.

Melissa had been to her ob-gyn, who diagnosed mild polycystic ovarian syndrome after listening to her history and checking an ultrasound; she recommended an ovulation-inducing medication. But Melissa had always preferred to do things in a more natural way, and wondered whether I could help her become pregnant without the use of drugs. "I know I can beef up my diet, and my girlfriend told me I should take some vitamins. I really want to give it a try; I'll do whatever you recommend."

I commended Melissa on the many good habits she had already developed, and on her strong and supportive relationship with her husband. Together, we agreed on a plan that included dietary changes (no high-glycemic-load carbohydrates—which you will learn more about in Chapter 3, "Nutrition"), several dietary supplements, guided imagery, and a daily thirty-minute walk rather than the more strenuous weekend hikes. I also asked Melissa to have regular sessions with an acupuncturist. She diligently followed my recommendations and five months later, she called me ecstatic with the news that she was pregnant.

In this chapter, I will review reproductive physiology and some of the most common deterrents to normal function. Even though many of you will have learned this information at some point, the details may not have stayed with you, and this knowledge is critical to your efforts at conception. Also, if you have been taking oral contraceptives for a long time, you may not know much about your cycles, as your underlying cycle is obscured by the effects of the pill. After I review the broad hormonal picture, I will help you determine when you are ovulating. Also in this chapter, I will discuss many of the lifestyle factors that impact this hormonal symphony, including your weight, exercise and sleep habits, and alcohol and nicotine intake.

Knowing Your Own Cycle: The Physiology

How do you view your menstrual periods? In American culture we often use derogatory language such as "the curse" or "I'm on the rag"; contrast this with traditional Chinese medicine, which refers to the menstrual period as "heavenly waters." Some women love to observe the cyclical nature of their bodies, watching them change throughout the month; other women feel "If I could eliminate this inconvenience from my life, I would be happy." Big Pharma has affirmed this message by creating birth control pills that allow you to have a period every three months, once per year, or not at all. Whatever your view is, I want you to become familiar with the basic physiology of your cycles.

A perfectly timed, complex hormonal cascade is responsible for the menstrual cycle. If you have normal, regular menstrual cycles—i.e., having a period every twenty-five to thirty-five days, with a duration of around five days—this is usually a good indication that much is right with your hormones, including those secreted by your hypothalamus, pituitary, thyroid, adrenals, pancreas, and ovaries. While the average-length menstrual cycle is twenty-eight days, normal ovulatory cycles vary from less than twenty-three days to more than thirty-five days.

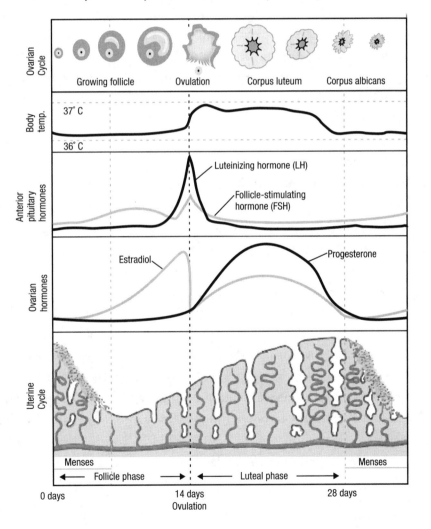

Physicians typically divide the cycle into two segments: the follicular and the luteal. The follicular phase begins on day 1, or the first day of menstrual blood, and runs up to the day you ovulate. The luteal phase begins the day after ovulation, and concludes the day before your next period begins. If your cycle was exactly twenty-eight days, the follicular phase (in which follicles are developing in the ovaries) would be days 1 to 14, and the luteal phase (when, after ovulation, the corpus luteum is formed from the follicle from which the egg was released) days 14 to 28. Ovulation would typically occur on day 14, and your period on day 28. Most women, however, do not have exact twenty-eight-day cycles, which is why it is a problem to assume that ovulation always occurs on the fourteenth day of the cycle. Keeping a diary will help you become familiar with your own cycle, and within a few months, you will be able to pinpoint your most fertile times. Please see the Basal Body Temperature Chart on pages 32-33.

The Follicular Phase

In response to the release of gonadotropin releasing hormone (GnRH) by your hypothalamus, the pituitary gland secretes FSH, or follicle-stimulating hormone, which stimulates the development of follicles in the ovary. The ripening follicles produce estrogen, and as estrogen levels rise, the lining of the uterus, or endometrium, becomes thicker. Up to twenty eggs start to mature in the follicles, and the cervix opens slightly, becomes softer, and rises higher up in the vagina.

When estrogen blood levels produced by the follicle reach a threshold, the pituitary gland produces a sudden surge of LH, or luteinizing hormone, and then a smaller surge of FSH. In response to these hormonal signals, ovulation begins within thirty-six hours. This hormonal surge is also what is detected by ovulation predictor kits. The surge leads the largest follicle to rupture and release its egg. Carried by fingerlike projections, the egg is moved from the ovary into the pelvic cavity and into the fallopian tubes. In conjunction with the rise in LH, your temperature will drop slightly. This marks the end of the follicular phase.

The Luteal Phase

After ovulation comes the luteal phase, when a woman's body prepares her uterus for implantation and pregnancy. The ruptured follicle, under the influence of LH, develops into the corpus luteum, which produces progesterone. Progesterone has several actions: it causes the endometrium to soften and thicken for implantation of the embryo, and it prevents developing eggs from being released from the other follicles.

When a fertilized egg burrows into the lining of the uterus, the cells that surround the egg begin to release another hormone, human chorionic gonadotropin (HCG). This hormone, unique to pregnancy (and indeed, the hormone measured in pregnancy tests), prevents the corpus luteum from regressing, thereby signaling the corpus luteum to stay alive beyond its normal sixteen days and continue producing progesterone to nourish the endometrial lining. As the outer cells of the fertilized egg are gradually transformed into the placenta, this structure produces progressively larger amounts of HCG. During the normal nonpregnant menstrual cycle, the nonfertilized egg and the corpus luteum die and progesterone levels drop, as does basal body temperature. In the absence of progesterone, the endometrium cells disintegrate and, together with the blood that has accumulated in the involuting uterine lining, slough—which is experienced as a menstrual period. The first day of menses marks the end of the luteal and the start of the next follicular phase.

The follicular phase begins with the onset of menses, and ends on the day of the luteinizing hormone (LH) surge. The luteal phase begins on the day of the LH surge, and ends at the onset of the next menses.

Basal Body Temperature Chart

Month: _____

Cycle Day	1	2	3	4	5	6	7	8	9	10	11	12	13	14	15	16	17	18
Day of Week																		
Time																		
Waking Basal Temp	99	99	99	99	99	99	99	99	99	99	99	99	99	99	99	99	99	99
	9	9	9	9	9	9	9	9	9	9	9	9	9	9	9	9	9	9
	8	8	8	8	8	8	8	8	8	8	8	8	8	8	8	8	8	8
	7	7	7	7	7	7	7	7	7	7	7	7	7	7	7	7	7	7
	6	6	6	6	6	6	6	6	6	6	6	6	6	6	6	6	6	6
	5	5	5	5	5	5	5	5	5	5	5	5	5	5	5	5	5	5
	4	4	4	4	4	4	4	4	4	4	4	4	4	4	4	4	4	4
	3	3	3	3	3	3	3	3	3	3	3	3	3	3	3	3	3	3
	2	2	2	2	2	2	2	2	2	2	2	2	2	2	2	2	2	2
	1	1	1	1	1	1	1	1	1	1	1	1	1	1	1	1	1	1
	98	98	98	98	98	98	98	98	98	98	98	98	98	98	98	98	98	98
	9	9	9	9	9	9	9	9	9	9	9	9	9	9	9	9	9	9
	8	8	8	8	8	8	8	8	8	8	8	8	8	8	8	8	8	8
	7	7	7	7	7	7	7	7	7	7	7	7	7	7	7	7	7	7
	6	6	6	6	6	6	6	6	6	6	6	6	6	6	6	6	6	6
	5	5	5	5	5	5	5	5	5	5	5	5	5	5	5	5	5	5
	4	4	4	4	4	4	4	4	4	4	4	4	4	4	4	4	4	4
	3	3	3	3	3	3	3	3	3	3	3	3	3	3	3	3	3	3
	2	2	2	2	2	2	2	2	2	2	2	2	2	2	2	2	2	2
	1	1	1	1	1	1	1	1	1	1	1	1	1	1	1	1	1	1
	97	97	97	97	97	97	97	97	97	97	97	97	97	97	97	97	97	97
	9	9	9	9	9	9	9	9	9	9	9	9	9	9	9	9	9	9
	8	8	8	8	8	8	8	8	8	8	8	8	8	8	8	8	8	8

Cycle Day	1	2	3	4	5	6	7	8	9	10	11	12	13	14	15	16	17	18
Circle Day of Intercourse	1	2	3	4	5	6	7	8	9	10	11	12	13	14	15	16	17	18
Describe Cervical Fluid																		
Cervix Hard/Soft																		
Cervix Position																		
Vaginal Sensation																		

Cycle Day	1	2	3	4	5	6	7	8	9	10	11	12	13	14	15	16	17	18
OPK Result																		
Pregnancy Test Result																		
Other Notes:																		
Poor Sleep																		
Alcohol																		
Illness																		
Additional Information:																		

Describe
Cervical Fluid: **E** = Eggwhite **C** = Creamy **S** = Sticky   *Cervix Hard/Soft:* **H** = Hard **S** = Soft

Vaginal Sensation: **D** = Dry **M** = Moist **W** = Wet   *Cervix Position:* **H** = High **M** = Middle **L** = Low

Cycle: _____

19	20	21	22	23	24	25	26	27	28	29	30	31	32	33	34	35	36	37	38	39	40
99	99	99	99	99	99	99	99	99	99	99	99	99	99	99	99	99	99	99	99	99	99
9	9	9	9	9	9	9	9	9	9	9	9	9	9	9	9	9	9	9	9	9	9
8	8	8	8	8	8	8	8	8	8	8	8	8	8	8	8	8	8	8	8	8	8
7	7	7	7	7	7	7	7	7	7	7	7	7	7	7	7	7	7	7	7	7	7
6	6	6	6	6	6	6	6	6	6	6	6	6	6	6	6	6	6	6	6	6	6
5	5	5	5	5	5	5	5	5	5	5	5	5	5	5	5	5	5	5	5	5	5
4	4	4	4	4	4	4	4	4	4	4	4	4	4	4	4	4	4	4	4	4	4
3	3	3	3	3	3	3	3	3	3	3	3	3	3	3	3	3	3	3	3	3	3
2	2	2	2	2	2	2	2	2	2	2	2	2	2	2	2	2	2	2	2	2	2
1	1	1	1	1	1	1	1	1	1	1	1	1	1	1	1	1	1	1	1	1	1
98	98	98	98	98	98	98	98	98	98	98	98	98	98	98	98	98	98	98	98	98	98
9	9	9	9	9	9	9	9	9	9	9	9	9	9	9	9	9	9	9	9	9	9
8	8	8	8	8	8	8	8	8	8	8	8	8	8	8	8	8	8	8	8	8	8
7	7	7	7	7	7	7	7	7	7	7	7	7	7	7	7	7	7	7	7	7	7
6	6	6	6	6	6	6	6	6	6	6	6	6	6	6	6	6	6	6	6	6	6
5	5	5	5	5	5	5	5	5	5	5	5	5	5	5	5	5	5	5	5	5	5
4	4	4	4	4	4	4	4	4	4	4	4	4	4	4	4	4	4	4	4	4	4
3	3	3	3	3	3	3	3	3	3	3	3	3	3	3	3	3	3	3	3	3	3
2	2	2	2	2	2	2	2	2	2	2	2	2	2	2	2	2	2	2	2	2	2
1	1	1	1	1	1	1	1	1	1	1	1	1	1	1	1	1	1	1	1	1	1
97	97	97	97	97	97	97	97	97	97	97	97	97	97	97	97	97	97	97	97	97	97
9	9	9	9	9	9	9	9	9	9	9	9	9	9	9	9	9	9	9	9	9	9
8	8	8	8	8	8	8	8	8	8	8	8	8	8	8	8	8	8	8	8	8	8

19	20	21	22	23	24	25	26	27	28	29	30	31	32	33	34	35	36	37	38	39	40
19	20	21	22	23	24	25	26	27	28	29	30	31	32	33	34	35	36	37	38	39	40

19	20	21	22	23	24	25	26	27	28	29	30	31	32	33	34	35	36	37	38	39	40

33

Identifying Your Most Fertile Time

Women are fertile for up to six days per cycle. The range is from five days before ovulation through the day of ovulation. It may surprise you to learn that your most fertile days are the two days *prior* to ovulation. This is because once released from its follicle, an egg survives somewhere between six and twenty-four hours. The longer fertile window is due to the ability of sperm to survive for up to five days in fertile cervical mucus. For pregnancy to occur, it is optimal to have intercourse *before* ovulation so that the sperm are close by and ready to fertilize the egg soon after it erupts from its follicle. During the fertile period, daily intercourse heightens the likelihood of conception.

The body provides multiple signs to point to your fertile window—however, unlike menses, the clues tend to be subtle. I hope you will enjoy observing your body and learning to predict when you are most likely to conceive. Alterations in the timing of your menstrual cycle and changes in your cervical mucus and in the position and feel of your cervix are some of the signs you will want to observe. A slight rise in your basal body temperature (BBT) just after you ovulate is another. You may also note a cramping pain in your pelvis, called *mittelschmerz,* when you ovulate. Finally, for folks who love technology, there is a high-tech option: you can purchase an ovulation predictor kit.

Timing Your Menstrual Cycle

You may already know that you have, for instance, an exact thirty-day cycle, month in and month out. A very regular cycle allows you to predict your fertile window by estimating the timing of ovulation based on the length of your previous cycles. When we calculate *backward,* the time between ovulation and the menstrual period is usually a relatively stable fourteen days; much more variable is the length of the pre-ovulatory or follicular phase. So for a regular thirty-day cycle, you would expect to ovulate on day 16, and this is one of the clues to estimating your fertile window. This method can be used in women with longer and shorter cycles, but is *unreliable* if your cycle length varies from month to month. If you have a shorter cycle of around twenty-three days, ovulation will likely occur around day 9. For a woman with a cycle lasting thirty-four days, ovulation does not occur until day 21 or so. (Some women do have short luteal phases, meaning they ovulate less than fourteen days before their periods. This shorter cycle can interfere with implantation and becomes a barrier to conception. More on this later in the chapter.)

Cervical Mucus

Cervical mucus changes over the course of your cycle. As estrogen levels rise during the follicular phase, the mucus produced by the cervix changes as well, making it more receptive to sperm. When you ovulate, the mucus has an abundance of salt, sugar, and amino acids, all of which are designed to facilitate the survival of sperm and their movement through the vagina and the cervix toward the egg. In this "hospitable" environment, sperm can survive for as long as six days. Most noticeable to the eye is that during ovulation, it changes from a scant amount of a sticky, opaque, whitish discharge to a transparent, glistening, slippery, and stretchy mucus. This is the point at which it is said to resemble egg white. Associated with the mucus is a sensation of wetness, slipperiness, or lubrication at the vulva.

When the mucus has maximal slippery and wet qualities, you are at your peak of fertility. This fertile cervical mucus typically lasts for three days, although it may last longer in younger women and be shorter in older women. After ovulation, progesterone, secreted by the corpus luteum, causes the mucus to change once again. It becomes scantier and whiter, loses its stretchiness, and actually impedes the survival of sperm and blocks it from passing through the cervix. When taking the pill, these changes are unlikely to occur, or they are much less obvious.

Assessing your cervical mucus is easily learned. If you wish to have an instructor, courses are available and include the Creighton Model FertilityCare System and the Billings Ovulation Method. The former has been studied in fifty couples with normal fertility. The study found that 76 percent of the couples using this method achieved pregnancy in their *first* month of trying.

Changes in the Cervix

Another way to tell when you are coming into your fertile stage is by noting changes in your cervix. While not everyone will be comfortable doing so, you can learn to examine your own cervix. With clean hands, squat down or place one foot on the toilet seat. Insert your middle finger deeply into your vagina until you touch the tip of your cervix. In general, fertility is indicated by a high, soft (think the consistency of your lips), open, and wet cervix. For most women (aside from health providers), this is unfamiliar territory, and these qualities are all relative. This means that it will probably take several cycles until you grasp the subtleties of your cervical changes. A dry, closed, firm (imagine the consistency of cartilage as in the tip of your nose), low cervix indicates the nonfertile stage. For women who have borne children already, you will notice that your cervix will always be a bit open and have more of an oval than a round shape. Once you get a sense of what a closed, firm cervix feels like, you can choose to check your cervix just one week a month. Begin when you first notice wet cervical fluid, and continue for a few days after you notice that your cervix is low, closed, and firm.

Basal Body Temperature

Basal body temperature (BBT) is another way to confirm ovulation. It refers to the rise in temperature of about 0.4 degrees Fahrenheit that typically follows ovulation and remains elevated for about fourteen days. Here's the catch: because it occurs just after ovulation, it is too late to use as a signal to predict that you are now in your fertile window. BBT *can* be used to help you learn your own pattern, which indicates when you will ovulate in the future.

To measure BBT, purchase a special BBT thermometer and take your temperature first thing in the morning before you sit up in bed, or eat or drink anything. (The BBT thermometer is much more accurate than a regular thermometer, and therefore is able to indicate tiny shifts in temperature.) After you chart your BBT for a few months, you can begin to predict when you will ovulate, based on the pattern you see from your temperature (for instance, your BBT rose around day 15 of your cycle).

Mittelschmerz and Other Clues

Some women notice cramping pain low in their abdomens at the time of ovulation, known as *mittelschmerz*. The pain can last for a few hours or for up to several days. Other women may have tender breasts associated with ovulation. Finally, some women notice midcycle spotting as a result of the drop in estrogen. Observing your own body and noting these signs can provide clues to when you are ovulating.

Ovulation Predictor Kits

Many women prefer high-tech options or find it confusing to figure out when they are ovulating. Ovulation predictor kits are widely available and can be very helpful. They measure the surge in LH that occurs up to thirty-six hours prior to ovulation. The upside of these kits is that they are quite accurate. The downside is that they identify a fairly narrow window of your total fertile time. Also, they are expensive and can have false positives, especially in women who have PCOS and/or who are over forty. Women who are forty-plus years sometimes have elevated LH levels; their follicles don't always respond to the LH surge, which the kit uses to predict ovulation. This means that although the kit may have accurately read the LH surge, in an older woman that does not definitively mean that the egg was released from its follicle.

A monitor that identifies a broader fertility window is the Clearblue Fertility Monitor. In addition to the LH surge, it measures a second hormone, estrone-3-glucuronide. This is a form of estrogen, which, as you now know, rises earlier in the follicular phase. Measuring the rise in estrogen helps identify the broader fertility window that begins four days prior to the LH surge. This extends the time that couples can plan to have intercourse to maximize their chances of conception.

There are some further tests that your physician can do in the office to detect ovulation. These include doing serial ultrasounds or checking blood levels of hormones. To summarize, the best clues that you can use at home are noticing fertile cervical mucus and a vulvar sensation of wetness.

A Note on Aging

As women age, their cycles change. While cycles typically show little variability between the ages of twenty and forty, after forty, menstrual cycles begin to shorten. This makes it more difficult to use cycle length as a tool for timing the fertile window. The normal hormone feedback loops work less well, and even with healthy estrogen levels, FSH levels rise as women age. Even regularly cycling women tend to have higher FSH levels at forty to forty-five compared with regularly cycling women aged twenty to twenty-four. Older women tend to have shorter follicular phases, which means the dominant follicle must mature more rapidly. The most significant change, however, is the aging of eggs. All of the eggs ever created in a woman's body are formed during her fetal life. And eggs age as women do. When a woman is twenty, they are twenty; at thirty, they have aged another decade, and so on.

Common Problems with Fertility

About 10 percent of couples have trouble with their fertility. It is usually advised that couples attempt to conceive for a year; 90 percent of couples will become pregnant within that time. If they are unsuccessful after a year, we begin to evaluate. The exception is, when the woman is over thirty-five, we begin to evaluate after six months—because aging is a concern.

In this section, I will describe the most common fertility problems in women as well as the major challenges in men. For women, a broad set of conditions leading to ovulatory dysfunction are most frequently found, followed by anatomical problems such as fibroids or blocked tubes; genetic issues are rarer. Ovulatory dysfunction can arise from disorders of the ovary itself, such as polycystic ovarian syndrome (PCOS); or secondary pituitary disorders leading to luteal phase dysfunction; elevated prolactin levels in blood; and abnormal thyroid function. Endometriosis, a disorder in which the tissue that normally lines the inside of the uterus grows outside the uterus, is another common cause of infertility.

Polycystic ovarian syndrome is the most common endocrine disorder causing infertility, affecting 5 to 10 percent of women of childbearing age. Symptoms of PCOS may show up at puberty with menstrual abnormalities, acne, and excessive facial and body hair. There is no single known cause of PCOS; it represents a mixed bag of endocrine and metabolic problems. Ovarian cysts, elevated insulin levels, and oxidative stress (an excess of free radicals, some of which are naturally created in the body; others are from environmental exposures) are all features of PCOS. There is a wide array of symptoms for PCOS; some women have very mild symptoms—facial hair, acne, slightly irregular periods that are easily controlled with diet and weight loss—while other women with PCOS have much more serious symptoms including the loss of ovulation, insulin resistance, and obesity. In Chapter 3, "Nutrition," I will review the anti-inflammatory diet, one example of a limited-carbohydrate diet shown to be successful in treating PCOS. Fertility is impaired in most women with PCOS, and miscarriages are more common as well.

In PCOS, the pituitary gland does not produce normal amounts of the hormones FSH and LH, and this results in disturbances in ovulation and menstruation. If the pituitary secretes more LH than FSH, the egg will not mature and there will be no menstrual cycle. This can lead to an excess of testosterone, which causes acne and unwanted hair growth. In addition, many women with PCOS either do not have a period or else have very light or erratic periods, along with infertility. Insulin resistance, where the receptors in the body no longer respond well (are resistant) to insulin, is another characteristic problem in PCOS. The body responds by producing even more insulin, but there still tend to be higher circulating levels of blood glucose and lower levels of sex hormone-binding globulin (SHBG). SHBG is a circulating protein that binds hormones, including testosterone and estrogen, which circulate in the bloodstream. When SHBG levels fall, the amount of free hormone in the blood, which is the biologically active form, is increased. Reduced amounts of SHBG means more circulating testosterone, causing excess facial hair, acne, and abnormal cholesterol and triglyceride levels. Insulin resistance can present physically as skin tags and/or skin darkening on the neck, armpit, or groin or a crease under the breasts, a manifestation called *acanthosis Nigricans*. Treatment usually requires a varied approach and can include weight loss, a low-glycemic-index diet, exercise, and sometimes pharmaceuticals ranging from birth control pills (if a woman does not wish to conceive) to ovulation inducers to insulin-sensitizing agents.

Luteal phase defect (LPD) is a disorder of the corpus luteum in which there is subnormal progesterone and estrogen production after ovulation, with a short (i.e., less than ten-day) luteal phase. This can result in abnormal uterine bleeding, infertility, and early pregnancy loss. Research studies are limited because LPD is neither well-defined nor easy to diagnose. The underlying problem is that the endometrium does not have sufficient time to mature because of inadequate progesterone (or an abnormal response to the progesterone) and a short phase. A study that followed recreational athletes (as opposed to elite athletes) over three menstrual cycles found that LPD was present as much as 79 percent of the time—46 percent inconsistently and 33 percent consistently. The disorder results in reduced FSH, blunted LH surge, decreased early follicular phase estradiol, and decreased luteal phase progesterone; the profile showed a hypometabolic state similar to what you would see in women who stop having their periods due to athletic activity. There was also a reduction of one thyroid hormone (T3) and insulin levels.

A short luteal phase can be diagnosed by finding an abnormal basal body temperature or low urinary progesterone level, or with an endometrial biopsy or ultrasound (this last one is the standard for the diagnosis of LPD). By following your own basal body temperature, you can assess the length of each part of your cycle and thereby measure your luteal phase. Dietary changes, backing off on exercise, traditional Chinese medicine (TCM) practices, and certain supplements can all help treat luteal phase disorder, as can intravaginal progesterone.

Another factor in infertility is *anatomical problems* such as fibroids, blocked tubes, an oddly shaped uterus, or blockages from infections such as chlamydia. Tubal blockage can be caused by scarring from pelvic surgery, STDs, or congenital defects. Fibroids, tumors, and endometriosis can also cause obstruction or ovarian or tubal damage. These anatomical problems are not typically seen during your regular doctor's visit for a pap smear. Should you experience difficulty conceiving, special imaging studies will be done to look for any such problems. Many anatomical issues can be successfully treated with surgery. For those that cannot, IVF may surmount the problem.

Ovulatory Infertility

Ovulatory infertility is responsible for between 20 and 40 percent of fertility problems in women, and can be caused by PCOS, hyperprolactinemia, excess stress, low thyroid levels, or endometriosis, although sometimes the etiology is unexplained. The type of treatment one receives depends on the reason for cessation of ovulation. Treatment may involve balancing sex hormones, thyroid hormones, or insulin levels. For women with ovulatory infertility, conventional medicine prescribes ovulation-inducing medications either orally or by injection.

Genetic issues are a final cause of infertility. Such factors include intersexed conditions, such as complete androgen insensitivity syndrome (AIS). Complete AIS is caused by a mutation in the androgen receptor, a protein on the cell's surface that normally responds to testosterone. Women with such a syndrome will not menstruate and cannot become pregnant because they have no uterus. Another condition is Turner's syndrome, which results from a missing or incomplete X chromosome. This syndrome may cause other problems beyond infertility, including heart defects and hypothyroidism. Genetic causes may also lead to male infertility presenting as either oligoasthenospermia (decreased sperm motility) or azoospermia (lack of sperm).

Male Fertility

While women are born with their lifetime supply of eggs, men's bodies are constantly making sperm—and male fertility depends on healthy sperm. To produce functional sperm, a man must produce sufficient testosterone and pituitary hormones to initiate and maintain sperm production in the testes. There must be enough sperm, of good motility and normal morphology (the sperm's shape and condition), to penetrate an egg (or ovum). In the testes, the hormone LH binds to receptor sites that turn on Leydig cells in the testicles, which stimulate testosterone production. FSH binds to receptors in the Sertoli cells in the seminiferous tubules, which stimulate the production of sperm—so that both sperm and testosterone production are stimulated by LH and FSH. It is worth noting that worldwide, sperm counts have been declining; reasons include environmental exposures and estrogen mimics, which are chemical compounds that abnormally attach to estrogen receptors and send inappropriate signals.

Lifestyle Factors and Fertility

As stated earlier, lifestyle factors can have powerful effects on our physiology as well as our ability to conceive. Some of these factors are a bit more complicated than they might seem at first blush. In this section I'll discuss the intricacies of how exercise, weight loss, smoking, and sleep impact fertility; and what you can do to improve your chances for conception.

Obesity

Obesity, defined as a BMI of over 30, is an important example of how normal physiology can be altered so that both fertility and your chances of having a healthy child are impaired. (Again, BMI is calculated by dividing weight in pounds by the square of height in inches, then multiplying this number by 703.) For example, PCOS is much more common in obese women. Even if they don't have PCOS, obese women are more often insulin-resistant and have higher levels of circulating insulin in their blood. Those elevated insulin levels interfere with the production of sex hormone-binding globulin (SHBG), which increases circulating androgens or male hormones. Lower SHBG also leads to increased conversion of the androgens into estrogen. In addition, obese women have higher estrogen levels in general, which deliver a negative feedback signal to the hypothalamic pituitary ovarian axis. Finally, the high insulin levels stimulate the production of abnormally high amounts of both testosterone and estrogen—these affect the pituitary and the pituitary regulating parts of the brain, and produce incomplete, or even complete, shutdown of the pituitary hormones that control the ovary.

Women who are obese and ovulate face infertility more frequently than do women who are of normal weight or overweight. In fact, many obese women don't ovulate at all, because stored body fat results in higher estrogen levels, which can obstruct ovulation. In particular, for every one BMI unit over 29 kg/m^2, a woman's likelihood of getting pregnant on her own drops 4 percent compared to a woman with a BMI between 21 and 29 kg/m^2. Obese men may have lower testosterone concentrations and erectile dysfunction, both of which can cause or contribute to infertility.

In addition, obesity has a direct effect on the developing egg. It appears that obesity alters the composition of follicular fluids, leading to higher levels of insulin, glucose, testosterone, and an important marker of inflammation, C-reactive protein. Obesity even interferes with ovulation that is induced by injections of HCG in assisted reproductive efforts. The altered fluid in the follicle affects the egg adversely, which in turn leads to greater difficulty in becoming pregnant, greater risk of early miscarriage, and poorer outcomes with IVF.

At this time, in the United States, population studies have found that at least one out of four women of reproductive age is obese. Even when obese women succeed in becoming pregnant, they are at increased risk of a number of complications, not only to the pregnancy but also to the health of the unborn child. Among these risks are a higher rate of miscarriage and preeclampsia (high blood pressure and protein in the urine after the twentieth week of pregnancy). Children born to obese women have an increased risk of being born with congenital anomalies, and as they grow older, a greater risk of obesity, of various kinds of heart disease, and diabetes. All of these factors underscore the importance of being within the normal weight range before becoming pregnant. Weight loss before pregnancy can help prevent all of these negative reproductive outcomes. The message here is that to have the healthiest child possible, you don't want to be obese when you conceive.

Exercise

Next, let's tackle exercise. If a woman is overweight, there is evidence from the Nurses' Health Study (one of the largest national studies of women's health, it began in 1976, expanded in 1989, and is now following 238,000 nurses) that when she exercises and loses weight, she will improve her chances of ovulation and subsequent fertility. On the other hand, women who are exceptionally athletic tend to have decreased fertility. Indeed, it is well-known that intense exercise in women leads to fertility problems. Researchers estimate that between 1 and 44 percent of all athletic women have amenorrhea, or a complete absence of menstrual periods. This is most prevalent in elite athletes in sports that emphasize being very thin, such as long-distance running or gymnastics; it is less common with bicycling and swimming. However, athletes of any kind tend to have higher rates of amenorrhea than the general population. A subtler problem, which athletic women experience intermittently, is a luteal phase defect.

More moderate physical activity has shown varying effects on fertility in different studies. The Nurses' Health Study revealed that there was less ovulatory infertility (which accounts for around one-fifth of all infertility) in women who exercised at least thirty minutes per day. In fact, each hour per week of vigorous activity was associated with a 7 percent lower relative risk of infertility. This was found to be important only in women who had not yet had any children. In those women, there was about one-third less ovulatory infertility. On the other hand, a survey of almost four thousand women showed that increasing the frequency, duration, or intensity of physical activity was associated with increased difficulty in conceiving. Women who exercised on most days had a 3.2 times higher risk of being infertile, while women who at any point exercised to exhaustion had a 2.3 times increased risk. These findings were independent of age, smoking, or BMI, and suggest that intensive exercise can interfere with a woman's fertility.

Interestingly, even during IVF, where a woman's reproductive physiology is completely overridden by prescribed hormones, women who reported exercising four hours or more per week for the past one to nine years were less likely to have live births. They were also three times more likely to experience cycle cancellation, and twice as likely to have implantation failure. Walking was associated with less risk than were more vigorous types of physical activity; women who walked one to three hours per week for ten to thirty years before IVF did not experience any change in outcome. However, four hours or more of exercise per week predicted that the IVF attempts were 50 percent less likely to be successful. Cardiovascular exercise had the most detrimental effect of all; when a woman exercised with a higher intensity than walking, there was a 30 percent lower chance of a successful pregnancy after the first IVF cycle.

While I would never want to tell women not to exercise, this is troubling information. When we play sports or exercise, it can disrupt our hypothalamic-pituitary-ovarian (HPO) axis. Excessive physical activity alters the release of GnRH from the hypothalamus, and also reduces FSH and LH, resulting in less ovarian stimulation and less estrogen. If the effect is mild, it can cause an intermittent luteal phase defect. If the activity involves strenuous exertion as well, there is also a chance that it will stimulate the hypothalamic-pituitary-adrenal (HPA) axis, leading to greater production of cortisol—which in turn activates the physiological stress response from the ovarian and adrenal axes. In well-trained athletes, the HPA has a milder response (i.e., the exercise is less stressful in a superb athlete). So if you play very competitive and intense sports, you might want to pull back on that activity before trying to conceive.

Male fertility is much less impacted by exercise. While it can result in changes in semen quality or sperm morphology, exercise does not seem to impair male fertility. The only time I might ask a man to curtail exercise is if he is extremely physically active and is having fertility problems.

In conclusion, the relationship between women's fertility and exercise is complicated. Moderate exercise is recommended, and probably helps; extreme exercise could impair conception. For an overweight woman, exercise is particularly important as part of her weight-loss plan and enhances fertility.

Smoking

Obstetricians are unanimous in telling their patients not to smoke while they are pregnant or trying to get pregnant. In many ways, the issue of giving up smoking is a no-brainer. I recognize that it is very hard to quit, but do consider these facts: population studies reveal that smoking makes it harder to get pregnant, requiring an average of two months longer than for nonsmokers. Smoking can damage the DNA in the chromosomes of both the developing egg and the sperm—and the more you smoke, the worse the damage. Chemicals in cigarette smoke accelerate follicular depletion and decrease the total number of eggs that are produced over a woman's lifetime, and women who smoke enter menopause on average two years earlier than nonsmokers, so the habit also shortens women's fertile years. A United Kingdom meta-analysis reviewed the data from twelve studies and revealed a 60 percent increased chance of infertility among women who smoke, and a 32 percent increased risk of failure if the woman attempts IVF. Nicotine can persist in the body for up to twenty days after its use. Yet these effects are reversible; several studies suggest that one year after you quit, your fertility returns to baseline levels.

When pregnant women smoke, the fetus receives even more nicotine than does the mother. Cigarette smoke contains more than four thousand different chemical compounds, including nicotine, tar, benzene, heavy metals, and carbon monoxide. Nicotine is fat-soluble and passes with ease across the placenta to the developing fetus. A meta-analysis showed that smoking during pregnancy was strongly associated with increased risk of placental abruption, ectopic pregnancy, and premature

45

rupture of the membranes. Smoking also contributes to intrauterine growth retardation, leading to low-birth-weight babies.

The scary saga continues after birth. If a pregnant woman smokes, it doubles the risk that her baby will experience sudden infant death syndrome. The children of women who smoke during pregnancy have higher rates of behavioral problems, anxiety, depression, ADHD, lowered IQ (a reduction of more than 4 points), lower socioeconomic status, and antisocial behaviors. And, in a woman who smokes one or more packs per day while pregnant, the likelihood her child will become a smoker later in life doubles.

While quitting smoking is certainly difficult, 46 percent of women who smoke at the time they conceive do successfully quit. A woman's quit rate is made more or less difficult by her partner's habit. If a woman lives with a partner who smokes, she is twice as likely to continue to smoke during pregnancy. Kudos to the male partner who quits smoking when his wife gets pregnant. He improves not only his own health but also his wife's, as well as the health of their unborn child.

Alcohol

Another behavior that affects your ability to have a baby is alcohol consumption. The Nurses' Health Study showed a positive association of ovulatory infertility in women who drank one or more drinks a day; less than one drink per day had no negative effect. One drink is defined as 0.6 ounces of pure alcohol. This is equivalent to 12 ounces of beer, 5 ounces of wine, 8 ounces of malt liquor, or 1.5 ounces or a "shot" of 80-proof distilled liquor (such as whiskey, rum, gin, or vodka). Other studies have showed mixed results—some revealing reduced fertility, others showing no effect at all. This, of course, is at low levels of alcohol intake.

Sadly, alcohol is more frequently abused by pregnant women than any other substance, and can cause fetal alcohol syndrome, which is characterized by intrauterine growth retardation; a variety of congenital defects; and abnormalities of facial development, the musculoskeletal system, and development of the brain. Children with fetal alcohol syndrome have lower intelligence, and this deficit persists throughout life. Three ounces of alcohol per day significantly increases the incidence of fetal alcohol syndrome; less than one ounce a day appears to have little or no increased risk. Six drinks per day increases the risk of a birth defect tenfold, to a 50 percent occurrence.

In men, chronic drinking is associated with lower testosterone levels, higher levels of sex hormone-binding globulin, elevated prolactin, the development of breast tissue (gynecomastia), erectile dysfunction, and higher levels of estradiol—in other words, drinking really messes up a man's sex hormones. Not surprisingly, this results in deterioration of sperm concentration, semen volume, and sperm motility. Following binge drinking, there is disruption of sperm production, and chronic drinking leads to narrowing of the seminiferous tubules as well as injury to the germinal epithelium, or innermost part of the testicles.

Alcohol also turns out to impact the success rate in IVF. A 2011 study in *Obstetrics and Gynecology* looked at 2,500 couples who underwent IVF. When both the man and the woman consumed more than four drinks per week, live birth rates were decreased by 21 percent; when only the female partner consumed more than four drinks per week, the live birth rate was reduced by 16 percent.

Sleep

More and more attention is being given to how sleep deprivation can affect health. Poor sleep has been linked to an increased risk for infection, cardiovascular disease, diabetes, obesity, cancer, and depression. And, according to the National Sleep Foundation, 70 percent of Americans don't get enough sleep. Sleep helps to recharge all of our organ systems—including the reproductive system. When we cut back on sleep, over time our relationships, mood, and immune function all suffer. Potential damage to fertility is incurred directly should our hormonal balance be altered, and indirectly when we resort to fertility-disrupting lifestyle factors such as caffeine overuse and weight gain.

Very few studies have been done on sleep deprivation and fertility, and the little information that we have is more suggestive than conclusive. Most of these studies have been performed on women who work shifts—especially nurses. In one study of sixty-eight nurses, 53 percent of the women noted menstrual changes resulting from working night shifts. The nurses reported that they slept one hour less on average, and took more time to fall asleep. In general, we know that working a night shift makes it harder to fall asleep, and results in poorer sleep, less total sleep, and less satisfying sleep altogether. Yet these results do not prove that shift work affects fertility. At this point, the evidence isn't entirely clear about exactly how sleep affects fertility.

An intriguing and under-researched piece of the sleep equation rests with circadian rhythms. This rhythm is our inner twenty-four-hour clock, and it is profoundly affected by light and darkness. The suprachiasmatic nucleus in the brain responds to signals from the retina, interprets them, and instructs another tiny gland—the pineal—to produce the hormone melatonin. Preliminary research from animal studies shows that more exposure to light increases LH and FSH secretion. This leads to seasonal breeding in animals, which we commonly notice with more animals being born in the spring. We humans supersede the seasons with artificial light, and have children any time of year. Still, the light connection may be important.

Light boxes have already shown promise in treating seasonal affective disorder (SAD) and depression. One study exposed volunteers to very bright light using light boxes of 3,000 Lux for three hours per day for three days; this increased secretion of LH, and suggests a possible strategy for treating women with abnormal luteal phases. A study in Russia exposed twenty-two healthy women ages nineteen to thirty-seven to either a bright light box or a dim light box, then crossed them over to the opposite exposure for their next cycle. Prolactin, LH, FSH, and ovarian follicle growth, as well as the likelihood of ovulation, were increased following the bright light exposure versus dim light.

A few suggestions follow to help you get the best possible night's rest:

- Attend to your circadian rhythms by keeping a regular sleep and awakening time, and by exposing yourself to bright morning light and to lower light in the evenings. Sleep in a completely dark room; make sure there are no blinking lights from TVs, computers, VCRs, etc. Some people find sleep masks and/or white-noise machines helpful.

YOUR BODY, YOUR LIFESTYLE, AND FERTILITY

- Avoid excess caffeine or alcohol, as they can either keep you from falling asleep or wake you up in the middle of the night.
- Don't eat a heavy meal late in the day, and avoid spicy or sugary foods four to six hours before bedtime.
- Do not exercise late in the day if this affects your sleep. Other overstimulating behaviors can include watching television or working on the computer. Instead, read a book that relaxes you, or listen to some quiet music.
- If you have difficulty falling asleep, use some of the mind-body techniques described in Chapter 6, "Mind-Body Medicine," such as the relaxing breath exercises, meditation, progressive muscular relaxation, self-hypnosis, and guided imagery. Alternatively, a calming tea such as chamomile or a warm bath before bedtime helps many people get to sleep. Aromatherapy with lavender can also help some drift off.
- Remember that you must "let go" into sleep, and that it is an act of surrendering daytime consciousness. If there are things you are worried about forgetting, keep a notepad next to your bedside for jotting down notes.

I opened this chapter by saying that if you have regular cycles lasting twenty-three to thirty-five days, you can assume that much is right with your hormones and likely with your fertility as well. For those of you who have irregular periods, a discussion with your doctor may be warranted to explore whether you have PCOS and what might be done about it. Another reason to consult your doctor is if you find that your BBT charts reveal a short luteal phase. Do continue moderate exercise; however, realize that extreme sports or vigorous exercise are an impediment when seeking to conceive. I hope that the information in this chapter will convince you, if necessary, to bring your weight within normal limits, to quit smoking, and to limit alcohol to one beverage per day when seeking to conceive. The evidence clearly supports a healthy respect for the power of lifestyle to enhance fertility!

CHAPTER THREE

NUTRITION

A thirty-one-year-old medical assistant whom I'll call Amanda came to see me for preconception advice. She said, "I want to get pregnant soon, but I don't feel like I'm in balance. I crave sugar, and am constantly trying to keep those feelings at bay. My other downfall is cheese. I like fish and seafood, but I don't eat them often. Lately I have tried to clean up the way I've been eating. I've added kale, and I've stopped drinking alcohol, which I realized I was using to help cope with stress." Amanda is typical of many young women who come to see me. They have some of the information they need, but not all; and sometimes they have fallen into bad habits.

For the sake of their unborn children, women are most motivated to make lifestyle adjustments when they are pregnant. Eliminating risky behaviors, so difficult at other times, becomes almost easy in service to the newly developing life. We are at our most altruistic, consciously setting aside our own needs and preferences for the sake of another.

In my practice, I often see an incredible shift in women's readiness to change, and confidence that they will succeed when they are preparing for pregnancy. Quitting smoking, exercising wisely, avoiding harmful environmental chemicals, and making dietary changes are all open for discussion. This turns out to be extremely valuable for men and women as they seek to enhance conception, carry pregnancy to term, and deliver a healthy baby.

Of all the ways you can influence your health, nutrition is the area where you have the most control. You may not be able to limit how much pollution you're exposed to; you can't always affect how much stress you're under (although in this book, I will suggest ways to reduce both); but you do have tremendous control over what you put into your mouth. In this chapter, I will show you the evidence for how your choices can improve your fertility. But first, I will outline the overall principles of eating for a lifetime of good health.

The Anti-Inflammatory Diet

The Mediterranean diet has been shown across multiple studies to be one of the healthiest ways to eat. It has been proven to reduce the risk of heart disease, cancer, diabetes, Alzheimer's, and even depression. And yes, it has been shown to increase fertility. The anti-inflammatory diet is a form of the Mediterranean diet. This isn't a "diet" per se, as it is not intended as a weight-loss program (although people often do lose weight on it), nor is it an eating plan to practice for only a limited period of time. Rather, it is a way of eating that helps your body maintain optimum health.

Inflammation is familiar to all of us. Consider how your skin responds with an inflammatory response to a mosquito bite; it becomes red, swollen, warm, and tender. It also itches, due to the histamines released. Inflammation is how your immune system fends off infections and promotes healing in response to injuries. It does so by secreting chemical messengers, which activate a healing response. Acute inflammation is useful and is the signal for the body to turn on healing responses; but chronic inflammation is a problem. This occurs when our immune systems don't turn off the inflammatory signals, even though there is nothing more to fight, thus damaging our own tissues. While we don't know all the reasons for chronic inflammation, an unhealthy diet, stress, obesity, and environmental toxins are all triggers. The anti-inflammatory diet alters the chemical messages produced by the body, and helps to modulate its responses, thereby improving overall health. Along with reducing chronic inflammation, this diet provides ample vitamins, minerals, essential fatty acids, dietary fiber, and phytonutrients.

The anti-inflammatory diet aims for variety and stipulates that food should be as fresh and as close to its natural form as possible. In addition, there are three major directives: increase the omega-3 fatty acids in the diet; eat lower-glycemic-load carbohydrates; and eat abundant vegetables and fruits, preferably organic.

Most women need to consume 2,000 calories or less a day in order to maintain a healthy weight. With the anti-inflammatory diet, you will be getting 40 to 50 percent of your calories from carbohydrates, 30 percent from fat, and 20 to 30 percent from protein. Attempt to include carbs, fat, and protein at every meal.

Below are the basic nutritional needs of an average woman, based on a 2,000-calorie-per-day diet:

Fats (600 calories per day, or 67 grams; ratio of 1:2:1 saturated to monounsaturated to polyunsaturated)
Consume: olives, avocados, nuts, extra-virgin olive oil
Avoid: fat in poultry or meats, products made with palm kernel oil, trans fats

Omega-3s and omega-6s
Consume: fresh or frozen wild salmon, canned sockeye, sardines, black cod, herring, omega-3 fortified eggs, walnuts, and freshly ground hemp and flaxseeds
Avoid: safflower and sunflower oils, corn, cottonseed, and mixed vegetable oils, and products made with them such as crackers and pastries; margarine, vegetable shortening, partially hydrogenated oils

Protein (50 to 80 grams per day)

Consume: low-mercury fish, high-quality cheese, omega-3 eggs, yogurt, beans, legumes, nuts, seeds, quinoa, and bulgar; small amounts of organic chicken and occasional lean meat that is organic and grass fed and finished

Avoid: meats in general and especially processed meats

Fiber (40 grams per day)

Consume: fruits, vegetables, whole grains, muesli and granola made with whole oats, nuts, seeds, flaxseed

Avoid: cereal with flour as first ingredient and low-fiber foods

Phytonutrients

Consume: fruits, vegetables, cruciferous vegetables (one per day), citrus fruits and cooked mushrooms

Avoid: raw mushrooms

Beverages

Consume: water and drinks that are mostly water, such as tea

Avoid: more than one cup of coffee or more than one alcoholic beverage per day; sodas

When you're pressed for time, it's easy to just pop into a fast-food restaurant, grab a bite, and go. However, most fast food is rich in unhealthy fats, low in vegetables and fruits, and loaded with high-glycemic-load carbs. In other words, it's the exact opposite of what's recommended in an anti-inflammatory diet. To enhance your fertility, you will want to eat more whole food and less processed and refined foods. You will want to be more thoughtful of who prepares your food, with whom you eat it, and how much of it you eat.

Sometimes, people can become so anxious about their diet that they're afraid to eat just about anything. And doctors may contribute to that fear because we talk mostly about the risks of consuming certain foods. Let me emphatically state that I believe eating is one of life's great pleasures. Eating healthfully can and should provide vast enjoyment. As you will see, an anti-inflammatory diet is neither overly restrictive nor devoid of flavors, textures, and tastes. You will probably notice, as you eat this way, that you feel better and have more energy. Subtle improvements in your health, such as a clearer complexion and reduced achiness, may also occur. This overall sense of well-being helps reinforce your new style of eating.

Sample Meal Plan for One Week of a Fertility Enhancing Anti-inflammatory Diet

Day 1: Breakfast: ¾ cup steel-cut oatmeal with cinnamon, cardamom, and ginger added when the cereal is half-cooked, then sprinkled with 1½ tablespoons freshly ground flaxseed, ½ cup freshly sliced mango or other fresh fruit, and ¼ cup walnuts. Add ½ cup organic whole milk; sweeten to taste with up to 1 tablespoon local honey.

Lunch: 1½ cups vegetarian chili with a green salad (2 cups spring mix with ½ medium tomato, ¼ cup chopped cucumber, ½ medium carrot, 2 tablespoons walnut oil, and ½ tablespoon balsamic vinegar).

Dinner: 4 ounces broiled wild salmon with ½ cup steamed cauliflower, ½ cup steamed carrots, and a small baked sweet potato.

Snack: 2 mandarin oranges and ½ cup organic whole-fat cottage cheese.

Total calories: 2048

Day 2: Breakfast: 1 cup cooked quinoa with ½ cup ricotta cheese, 1½ tablespoons ground flaxseed, ¼ cup dried apricots, and 2 tablespoons cranberries; sweeten to taste with up to 1 tablespoon local honey.

Lunch: ¾ cup brown rice, ½ cup black beans, and ½ cup mixed steamed veggies with ½ medium avocado.

Dinner: 1 cup homemade vegetable soup, 4 ounces broiled wild Alaskan halibut, and ½ cup roasted Brussels sprouts.

Snack: small smoothie made with frozen fresh fruit (½ cup frozen strawberries, 1 banana), ½ cup organic plain yogurt, ½ cup soy milk, and ice.

Total calories: 1995

Day 3: Breakfast: 8 ounces Greek (full-fat) yogurt with ¼ cup almonds, 1 cup fresh raspberries and blackberries, and 1½ tablespoons flaxseed.

Lunch: 4 ounces baked organic chicken with ½ cup roasted broccoli florets and ¾ cup quinoa.

Dinner: 1½ cups vegetarian masala dish with ½ cup garbanzo beans over ¾ cup wild rice.

Snack: 1 cup whole olives with ¼ cup crumbled feta cheese and 1 cup edamame (can be spread throughout the day).

Total calories: 1962

Day 4: Breakfast: 2 omega-3–enriched eggs cooked as a frittata with 1 ounce cheese, ½ roasted red bell pepper, ¼ cup steamed chopped asparagus, and ¼ cup mushrooms.

Lunch: large mixed salad (2 cups spinach, ½ cup kidney beans, 2 tablespoons sunflower seeds, ½ cup chopped green apple, and 2 ounces organic cheddar cheese) with up to 2 tablespoons of vinaigrette salad dressing.

Dinner: 1 cup cooked quinoa pasta with ½ cup arugula, ½ cup kalamata olives, 2 ounces mozzarella cheese, 1 tablespoon olive oil, and 4 cloves crushed garlic.

Snack: ½ cup blueberries and one small square of 70 percent dark chocolate.

Total calories: 1738

Day 5: Breakfast: ¾ cup steel-cut oatmeal with cinnamon, cardamom, and ginger added when the cereal is half-cooked, then sprinkled with ¼ cup chopped pecans, 1½ tablespoons freshly ground flaxseed, and ½ cup fresh organic strawberries. Add ½ cup organic whole milk; sweeten to taste with up to 1 tablespoon local honey.

Lunch: vegetarian Cobb salad (2 cups spring mix, ¼ cup sliced radishes, ½ cup cherry tomatoes, ¼ cup diced cucumber, 1 omega-3–enriched hard-boiled egg, ½ medium avocado, and 2 tablespoons organic green goddess dressing) sprinkled with ¼ cup roasted soy beans.

Dinner: 4 ounces broiled sablefish, ¾ cup sautéed oriental vegetables (bok choy, napa cabbage, onion, broccoli, and carrots), and ½ cup steamed black or wild rice.

Snack: ¾ cup Greek (full-fat) yogurt with ½ cup blueberries, drizzled with local honey and ¼ cup walnuts.

Total calories: 1958

Day 6: Breakfast: 1 cup Greek (full-fat) yogurt with ¼ cup almonds, 1 cup fresh fruit, and 1½ tablespoons flaxseed sprinkled on top. One organic apple sliced and spread with 2 tablespoons cashew butter.

Lunch: grilled Portobello mushroom topped with ½ roasted red bell pepper and 1 slice organic provolone cheese. One heirloom tomato, sliced and drizzled with 1 tablespoon olive oil and chopped fresh basil, and one slice of multigrain bread.

Dinner: 4 ounces tofu and Asian vegetable stir-fry served over 1 cup steamed brown rice.

Snack: vegetable crudité (2 medium carrots sliced, 1 small head of endive, 3 radishes) with ½ cup hummus.

Total calories: 2012

Day 7: Breakfast: 2 omega-3–enriched eggs cooked as an omelet with ¼ cup sautéed onion, ½ cup spinach, ¼ cup sliced mushrooms, and ¼ cup shredded mozzarella cheese.

Lunch: pasta salad (1 cup cooked quinoa pasta, 2 cloves of garlic, ¾ cup broccoli florets sautéed in 2 tablespoons olive oil, sprinkled with 2 ounces feta cheese and 2 tablespoons pine nuts) with 2 tangerines.

Dinner: 1½ cups black-bean and kale soup with mixed greens salad (1 cup spring mix, 1 chopped medium green apple, and 1 ounce organic cheddar cheese) topped with 1 tablespoon walnut oil and ½ tablespoon apple cider vinegar.

Snack: 1 cup organic raspberries and 1 small square of 70 percent dark chocolate.

Total calories: 1966

Carbohydrates

On the anti-inflammatory diet, you'll want to get most of your carbs in the form of less refined, less processed foods with a low glycemic index and load. Glycemic index, or GI, is a measure of how rapidly carbohydrates are metabolized into blood sugar in the body. Glycemic load is a more sophisticated calculation that assesses how much of the food is actually carbohydrate. For example, carrots with a high glycemic index of 71 are primarily fiber, thus their glycemic load is a low 6. High-glycemic-load foods include doughnuts at 76, pretzels at 81, and instant rice at 87.

It's much healthier to eat lower-glycemic-load carbs that are more slowly metabolized than high-glycemic carbs that are quickly metabolized. When you eat high-glycemic carbs, your body responds by producing more insulin to control your blood sugar. Physiologically, this has several adverse consequences. Elevated insulin is followed by the production of more insulin-like growth factor one, which increases inflammation and the risk of cancer and impairs fertility. Eventually, it leads to insulin resistance, which over time leads to diabetes, metabolic syndrome, and heart disease.

With respect to fertility, elevated insulin levels also lead to decreases in sex hormone-binding globulin (SHBG). As noted earlier, SHBG's main function is to bind hormones, including testosterone and estrogen, which circulate in the bloodstream. But SHBG has a preference for testosterone, and if SHBG is reduced, there is less bound and more free testosterone—which can interfere with conception. (In PCOS, a primary problem is elevated levels of male hormones including testosterone.) So eating a lot of pastries, white bread, fast food, and other high-GI products can actually reduce your chances of conceiving.

Do cut way back on foods made with wheat flour and sugar—at most, eat a sandwich on a baguette or breakfast cereal only once or twice a week. Stop eating altogether (or save for a rare occasion) chips, crackers, cookies, pretzels, and the like. And do eat more whole grains, such as steel-cut oatmeal, brown rice, quinoa, and wheat berries, in which the grain is largely intact. Don't be fooled by labels that claim to be whole-wheat-flour products, which have roughly the same glycemic load as those containing white flour.

When you prepare pasta, cook it al dente and eat it in moderation. Pasta has a moderate effect on blood sugar and need not be avoided entirely. In addition, eat more beans, winter squashes, and sweet potatoes. As much as possible, avoid all foods made with high-fructose corn syrup. A wonderful set of cookbooks that focus on glycemic load is *The Glucose Revolution, The Low GI Handbook,* and *The Low GI Cookbook.*

Fats

In terms of fats, out of 2,000 calories a day, 600 can come from fat (approximately 67 grams). Fat intake should be in a ratio of 1:2:1 saturated to monounsaturated to polyunsaturated fat. The terms *saturated, monounsaturated,* and *polyunsaturated* have to do with biochemistry, and they have very different impacts on health.

The classic saturated fats are butter, other full-fat dairy products, and the fat in chicken or meat. The U.S. Department of Agriculture's Center for Nutrition Policy and Promotion 2011 Dietary Guidelines for Americans recommends that we limit saturated fat to less than 10 percent of our total calories. Most Americans do not come close to meeting this guideline and need to cut back. Do a personal assessment (see Chapter 2) and determine whether you need to reduce your intake of saturated fat by eating less butter, cream, unskinned chicken and fatty meats, and products made with palm kernel oil.

It turns out that the healthiest class of fats are monounsaturated, which include the fat in olives, avocados, and nuts, especially walnuts, cashews, and almonds, and butters made from these nuts. Extra-virgin olive oil is primarily a monounsaturated oil, and is my preferred choice for most cooking. When you need a neutral-tasting oil, use organic expeller-pressed canola oil (also primarily monounsaturated).

Polyunsaturated fats include the essential category of fats, omega-3 and omega-6. They are termed *essential* because we cannot form them ourselves and therefore must consume them in our diets. Both are necessary for optimal health. Omega-6 initiates inflammation in our bodies, and omega-3 has an anti-inflammatory component. We need both, and in the right proportions. In the United States, we get far too much omega-6 and not enough omega-3 in our diets. Ideally, we should be consuming a ratio of 2:1 omega-6 to omega-3, but in the SAD, or Standard American Diet, it's often 20:1 of omega-6s to omega-3s.

Inflammation is an underlying root cause of many illnesses, including Alzheimer's, ulcerative colitis, various cancers, and heart disease. There even appears to be a relationship between inflammation and depression; for example, there is more depression in countries with lower fish consumption (and therefore more inflammation), including the United States, Germany, and Canada (as opposed to Japan). In Iceland, located in the cold, dark north, where you might expect there to be much higher incidents of depression, the population consumes so much omega-3 that they actually have very low rates. Several studies have also shown that women can help prevent postpartum depression by loading up on their omega-3s prior to giving birth.

Because the two classes of omegas are broken down by the same enzymes, in effect, they are competing for the enzymes. The net result is that to balance the scale, many of us need to not only increase omega-3s but also reduce our omega-6s. If you eat fish several times a week but also consume a lot of omega-6, you'll still tend toward a pro-inflammatory state. Reduce omega-6 by avoiding safflower and sunflower oils, corn, cottonseed, and mixed vegetable oils, as well as processed foods made with them (such as crackers and pastries). Similarly, avoid margarine, vegetable shortening, and any products that contain them, as well as products with any type of

NUTRITION

partially hydrogenated oils. These partially hydrogenated oils are a source of trans fats in the diet, which are also pro-inflammatory and have been shown to impair fertility.

While we need them in order to be healthy, it is relatively difficult to find sufficient sources of omega-3 fatty acids in American diets. The best sources are salmon (preferably fresh or frozen wild, or canned sockeye); sardines packed in water or olive oil; black cod (sablefish or butterfish); herring; omega-3–fortified eggs; walnuts; and hemp and flaxseeds (be sure to grind them fresh before eating). In Chapter 4, "Supplements," I will discuss the use of fish-oil supplements as another strategy to get the omega-3s that you need.

Protein

Protein is the third macronutrient in our diets (in addition to fats and carbs). You should consume 50 to 80 grams per day on a 2,000-calorie diet; less if you have liver or kidney problems, allergies, or autoimmune disease. Proteins are not all alike. Animal proteins come with more saturated fat and cholesterol, and are linked to higher rates of cancer. They also appear to impair fertility. In general, eat more vegetable and less animal protein. The exceptions are fish, eggs, and yogurt. Beans, legumes, nuts, and seeds provide abundant amounts of vegetable protein. Even grains contain protein, with quinoa, amaranth, and bulgur being particularly rich sources.

Fiber

Most of us need more fiber in our diets—ideally 40 grams per day. Fruits are a good source, especially berries, as are vegetables and whole grains. Breakfast cereals such as muesli and granola made with whole oats, nuts, and seeds can also be good sources of fiber. However, most other cereals should be avoided, as they are high-glycemic-load sources of flour and sugar. Avoid any cereal that has flour (including whole wheat flour) as the first ingredient. And cereal should provide at least 5 grams of fiber per 1-ounce serving.

Phytonutrients

Phytonutrients are another important component of the anti-inflammatory diet. You get them by eating a wide variety of fruits, vegetables, and mushrooms. Ideally,

61

choose fruits and vegetables of all colors, especially berries, tomatoes, orange and yellow fruits, and dark leafy greens, to get maximum protection against age-related diseases (including cardiovascular disease, cancer, and neurodegenerative disease).

One class of vegetables and one class of fruits deserve special mention. Cruciferous vegetables alter the metabolism of estrogen to safer forms. Ideally, and especially when preparing for pregnancy, attempt to eat a crucifer each day (broccoli, Brussels sprouts, cauliflower, cabbage). Citrus fruit is a rich source of bioflavenoids, which improve circulation and blood flow, including that going to the uterus.

Safe, Clean Foods

Whenever you can, eat organic, and avoid conventionally grown crops that are most likely to carry pesticide residues. I know that eating organic can be expensive. To help determine which vegetables and fruits should be eaten only organic and which of the conventionally grown are okay, the President's Cancer Panel has put together lists of the Dirty Dozen and the Clean 15 fruits and vegetables. The Dirty Dozen tested positive for at least forty-seven and up to sixty-seven chemicals. It is better to avoid the Dirty Dozen completely if organic is unavailable. While the list varies a bit from year to year, usually it includes celery, peaches, strawberries, apples, domestic blueberries, nectarines, sweet bell peppers, spinach, kale, collards, cherries, potatoes, imported grapes, and lettuce.

On the other hand, the produce on the Clean 15 list had few pesticide residues. You can eat these in nonorganic form, thus avoiding the extra cost of organic. Typically the Clean 15 includes onions, avocados, sweet corn, pineapples, mango, sweet peas, asparagus, kiwi, cabbage, eggplant, cantaloupe, watermelon, grapefruit, and sweet potatoes. You can find the list at www.ewg.org.

Another benefit of organic is that the food cannot contain genetically modified organisms (GMOs). We do not have conclusive evidence that GMO foods are risky to humans. However, most countries around the world have banned production due to health and environmental concerns. To be on the safe side, I believe it is worth avoiding GMO foods. This is a difficult recommendation to follow in the United States, as the government does not require labeling of GMO food. Since an estimated 91 percent of the soy, 88 percent of canola, and 90 percent of sugar beets produced in the United States use GMO technology, buying organic is the most practical way to avoid GMOs.

Beverages

Beverages also factor into an anti-inflammatory diet. Drink water or drinks that are mostly water (tea, very diluted fruit juice, or sparkling water with lemon), and use a filter at your tap to remove the chlorine. I will tell you more about filters and water safety in the environmental chapter.

In general, tea is preferable to coffee and has been linked to better fertility; especially enjoy good-quality white, green, or oolong tea. However, if you love your one cup of coffee in the morning, go ahead and have it. If you drink alcohol, be sure to limit your intake to one 5-ounce glass of wine per day or one 12-ounce beer.

Nutrition and Fertility

Now that I have laid out the basics of the anti-inflammatory diet, I will review the research on diet and fertility. One study that I will frequently refer to is the Nurses' Health Study II (NHS). This study was initiated by Dr. Walter Willett from the Harvard School of Public Health in 1976, then expanded in 1989. It followed a group of 18,555 married nurses, including a subset of women who indicated that they were trying to conceive. Food-frequency questionnaires were added to the study in 1991 and completed every four years. This is a common nutrition research tool in which participants indicate the frequency with which they consume various foods. Dr. Willett's team devised a scoring system based on dietary and lifestyle factors, such as fat intake, alcohol consumption, and frequency of exercise, and correlated them with the frequency with which the woman experienced ovulatory infertility. The NHS found 438 women with ovulatory infertility, which causes 30 percent of fertility problems.

Overall, the women with the best fertility diet scores, and therefore the lowest risk for infertility, ate less trans fat and sugar, more protein from vegetables than from animals, and more fiber and iron; took more multivitamins; had lower body mass

63

indexes; exercised for thirty minutes each day; and, surprisingly, consumed more high-fat dairy products and less low-fat dairy products. Regardless of age or prior pregnancy, the relationship between a higher fertility diet score and a lower risk for infertility remained similar.

Trans fats and Fertility

Interestingly, of all the fats, only trans fats played a role in ovulatory infertility in the NHS study. At the turn of the twentieth century, industries discovered how to give fats a long shelf life by adding hydrogen atoms to them, then twisting the fats into an artificial (or in biochemistry terms *trans*) configuration. This process creates fats that are partially hydrogenated. *Partially hydrogenated vegetable oils are used in commercial baked goods because these oils are cheaper than butter, and produce foods that take a very long time to spoil.*

The NHS found that each 2 percent increase in calories from trans fats, as opposed to carbohydrates, was associated with a 73 percent greater risk of ovulatory infertility. Obtaining 2 percent of energy intake from trans fats rather than from polyunsaturated fats was associated with a similar increase in risk. In addition, obtaining 2 percent of energy from trans fats rather than from monounsaturated fats was associated with a more-than-doubled risk. Thus, the researchers concluded that consuming trans fats drastically increases the risk of ovulatory infertility when eaten instead of carbs, or monounsaturated and polyunsaturated fats.

Trans fats have two mechanisms by which they disrupt fertility. They increase inflammation in the body, which interferes with ovulation, conception, and early embryonic development. In addition, trans fats have been shown to stop the activation of PPAR-gamma, hormone receptors that affect insulin sensitivity. The average amount of trans fats in Americans' diets halves PPAR-gamma activity, resulting in higher circulating insulin.

Pay attention to packaging. If there is less than 0.45 percent trans fats per serving, a company can claim that there are *no* trans fats. However, a typical small bag of potato chips contains four servings; if you eat the whole bag, you could be consuming a significant amount of trans fats, even though the bag may have been labeled as having none. Given the results of the NHS, it's best to studiously avoid trans fats while trying to conceive. The most effective way to do so is to eliminate foods that contain partially hydrogenated oils.

Protein and Fertility

Protein had a significant effect in the NHS; adding one serving per day of red meat, chicken, or turkey increased the risk of ovulatory infertility by nearly one-third. In contrast, adding one serving of fish or eggs did not alter the risk, and adding one serving per day of vegetable protein protected against infertility. If animal protein was eaten instead of carbs, the risk of infertility was increased by nearly 20 percent. Swapping 25 grams of plant protein for the same amount of animal protein led to a 50 percent lower risk of ovulatory infertility.

A 140-pound person needs only 50 grams of protein a day, but in developed countries, people tend to consume far more than they need. In the NHS, the lowest protein intake was around 77 grams per day; the highest, 115 grams. Women in the highest intake group were 41 percent more likely to have ovulatory infertility than those in the lower-protein group, and those eating the most animal protein were 39 percent more likely to have infertility. Women with the highest intake of plant protein were much less likely to be infertile. This is why I encourage my patients to consume generous portions of beans, nuts, and legumes when they are trying to conceive.

Another good reason to switch over to plant protein relates to environmental issues. Animal husbandry practices can be pretty horrendous, from both ethical and health perspectives. For example, cows are ruminants, meant to eat grass. When they are fed corn, it often causes stomach infections, which are treated with high doses of antibiotics. In fact, the U.S. Food and Drug Administration confirmed that animal agriculture consumes 80 percent of all antibiotics used in the United States. The beef from these grain-fed feedlot animals has significant amounts of omega-6, as opposed to the meat from grazing animals, which provides more balanced amounts of omega-6s and omega-3s. In addition, these large animals bio-accumulate a lot of pesticides.

Read labels at the grocery store carefully. Grass-fed is not enough; all cows graze at some point in their lives. *Natural* has no standard meaning, and is actually just a marketing term. Ideally, look for a label that says *organic and grass-finished*. Alternatively, buy your meat at a farmers' market where you can speak with the farmer and hear how he raised his animals.

One of my colleagues, Mary Beth Augustine, has been a nutritionist at the Beth Israel Center for Health and Healing in New York City for eleven years. She has a fascinating story about how changing her diet led to better health and fertility:

In 1989, when I was twenty-two years old, I was diagnosed with Hodgkin's disease. I had six cycles of chemotherapy. I chose the type of chemo that could put me into menopause, because the alternate choice was potentially toxic to my heart. Unfortunately, freezing eggs wasn't an option back then. I finished my treatments in September 1990, and went into menopause within a year.

From 1991 to 1997, I had no periods at all, and I began to have horrible hot flashes and other symptoms. At age twenty-eight, I got married, and in December 1997, I saw a fertility specialist at Cornell in New York because I wanted to know if I could get pregnant. My follicle stimulating hormone levels—the hormone that stimulates an egg follicle to grow every month—were elevated. I wasn't having periods either, so they said I had a less than 1 percent chance of conceiving.

My hot flashes were increasing, and I wanted to treat them naturally, rather than using hormone replacement therapy. I began treating myself with 120 mg of phytoestrogens, using isoflavones from soy foods such as tofu, miso, tempe, edamame, and roasted soy beans, and also flax. I started this regimen in January 1998, and soon my hot flashes disappeared, and my sleep quality and seasonal affective disorder got better as well.

After four months on the soy, in May 1998, I suddenly began having mood swings again, and my breasts became very tender. I came out of the shower crying one day and told my husband, "I'm going to have to go on hormones." He tried to reassure me, but I was very upset. I told my mom and a close girlfriend, and they both said, "I think you're pregnant." I thought they were crazy, but I took a pregnancy test and sure enough, it indicated that I was! I could hardly believe it; I went back to Cornell, and they confirmed that my HCG level (human chorionic gonadotropin, the hormone produced by a developing embryo) was through the roof. My husband and I were elated.

I had my first daughter in the fall. I breast-fed her for two years, and when I stopped, I had my period. I decided to try to conceive again. We became pregnant with our second daughter. I truly feel that it was due to the soy regimen that I was able to conceive.

Given Mary Beth's personal experience with soy, she sometimes recommends it to her clients, introducing it after three months' trial of a gluten-free diet. The first month, she recommends one serving a day; the second month, two servings per day; the third month, three servings per day. She asks her patients to observe whether there are changes in cervical mucus or menstrual cycle. On the other hand, for her vegetarian patients who are eating soy two or three times a day, she might suggest the opposite and eliminate soy if they have ovulatory infertility, menstrual problems, or hormonal issues.

Approximately 3 percent of women with unexplained infertility have celiac disease. Since this is entirely corrected by eating a gluten-free diet, a trial period off all gluten is warranted. Soy foods are more complex. A plant protein, soy is a rich source of phytoestrogens or plant-based estrogen. These phytoestrogens are much weaker than our naturally circulating estrogen. In a woman who is deficient in estrogen, as Mary Beth was, adding soy might help correct the problem. On the other hand, we are exposed to an abundance of estrogens in our environment, and other women might do better to restrict soy. Unfortunately, there are neither research studies nor explicit symptoms to direct who will benefit from which piece of advice, so you will need to experiment on yourself or turn to your clinician for guidance.

Carbohydrates and Fertility

The Nurses' Health Study found that carbohydrates have a complex effect on ovulatory infertility. While the *total* amount of carbs was not found to be related to infertility, the *type* of carbs were, as noted earlier. In the study, a woman was 92 percent more likely to have ovulatory infertility if she was eating a lot of high-glycemic-load foods. The worst carb culprit was breakfast cereal, which showed a statistically significant negative effect on fertility (statistical significance means that the probability of obtaining that result merely by chance is less than 5 percent). Often we think of breakfast cereal as a healthy choice, particularly when the label proclaims it to be a "heart healthy" source of whole grain. However, what you're eating is primarily sugar, flour, and salt. Cereal companies devised a tricky way of dividing up the various sugars so that sugar isn't the first ingredient you read—often you'll see cane sugar, honey, fructose, high-fructose corn syrup, and molasses listed separately, as David Kessler points out in *The End of Overeating*. But if you combine all the ingredients in these types of labels, up to one-third of the cereal is sugar.

Mary Beth Augustine recommends a diet that is very similar to the one I have outlined in this chapter. In her practice, she has also found hidden gluten intolerance as another factor to watch for. While I recommend blood tests for celiac disease for women having trouble conceiving, Mary Beth has found that for women who test negative but have multisystemic symptoms such as joint pain, rashes, digestive problems, PCOS, endometriosis, irritable bowel syndrome, or thyroid issues, it is good to go gluten-free for three months. She also recommends a gluten-free diet to women with a personal or family autoimmune history. If the gluten-free diet lessens any of the above symptoms, she suggests that her patient stay on the restricted diet.

Antioxidants, Vitamins, and Fertility

Consuming vegetables and fruits is the best way to get antioxidants, which are a critical part of an overall anti-inflammatory diet. Antioxidants are especially important in male fertility, yet 80 percent of American men don't get the recommended five servings of fruits and vegetables per day.

Multivitamins are one way to address the shortages; however, they cannot match the benefits of adding more vegetables and fruits daily. Whenever possible, I strongly recommend that people eat healthful, whole foods, rather than take supplements. We are sometimes led to believe that once we discover the nutrient in a whole food, we can substitute a supplement (in this case, multivitamins for vegetables and fruits). Time and again, this has not proven to be true. It is a reductionist mind-set that equates a single component with the beneficial effects of the whole food.

Dairy and Fertility

Another surprising finding in the Nurses' Health Study was the different effects of drinking whole-fat versus low-fat milk. As a society, we commonly believe that low- or nonfat dairy is healthier than whole milk. However, this does not appear to be true if you're trying to conceive. The Nurses' Health Study showed that women who drank two or more servings a day of low-fat milk were more likely to be infertile than women who drank less than one serving per week. In fact, the women drinking more low-fat milk experienced an 85 percent greater chance of being infertile. Furthermore, women who had one or more servings per day of high-fat dairy were 27 percent *less likely* to be infertile than those who consumed less than one serving per week of low-fat dairy.

This may seem contrary to everything we've been told about dairy consumption. We tend to be concerned about the saturated fats in dairy; however, what most of us don't realize is that when the dairy companies remove the fat from milk, they alter its hormonal content. To prepare low-fat and nonfat dairy, whole milk is spun at high speeds to separate the fat from the water. Hormones separate differently according to their preference for fat. Estrogen and progesterone prefer fat, so that when milk is being separated, those hormones go into that layer. Androgens, insulin-like growth factor one (IGF-1), prolactin, and male hormones prefer the watery layer—hence a glass of low-fat milk gives you more male hormones and fewer female hormones. Prolactin is the hormone that induces milk production after childbirth; it also helps prevent you from getting pregnant when you're breast-feeding, and it is present in greater amounts in skim milk. IGF-1 decreases sex hormone binding globulin, thus resulting in more circulating testosterone—another fertility zapper.

If this were not problematic enough, consider what is added back into skim milk once it's separated. Skim milk usually has a bluish tint, which the dairy companies feel is unappealing to consumers. Usually they add either nonfat milk powder or

69

whey protein to get rid of the blue color. There is evidence that when animals' diets are enriched with whey protein, its androgenic effects decrease fertility.

Another important milk consideration is that in the United States, we milk pregnant cows very far into gestation. This is not traditional milking practice, but for the most part, farmers in this country are trying to maximize profits from their cattle. Since cows are mammals, when they advance in pregnancy, they have a lot of hormones circulating in their milk; this is perfectly "natural" for all mammals, but does not make for an ideal beverage for humans. Even organic dairies tend to milk the cows deep into pregnancy. One great source of information about milking practices is Cornucopia.org, which rates dairies. Some states don't have a single dairy that follows the better organic dairy-farming practices.

An alternative to cows' milk is goats' or sheep's milk products. Animal husbandry practices are not (yet) a problem for these animals. While not everyone likes the taste of goats' milk, the cheeses from it and sheep's milk are delicious and widely available. You'll also have an easier time finding healthier yogurts made from goats' and sheep's milk because yogurt is easier to ship.

Coffee and Other Drinks

Now that we've addressed milk, let's talk about its frequent companion, coffee. Many women believe that they have to completely stop drinking coffee when they are trying to get pregnant, but actually the data is mixed. This is because drinking coffee improves insulin sensitivity, so for example, women with PCOS or diabetes actually benefit from drinking some coffee. Many of us really enjoy our morning cups of joe, and the evidence just isn't there to recommend going off it entirely when trying to conceive.

My main concern about coffee is that some people use it as a stimulant because they don't get enough sleep. In order to function, often they tank up during the day. Caffeine has a long half life (the amount of time it takes half of it to clear from your body); too much in the morning or throughout the day means that you will still have caffeine on board when it is time to go to sleep. If you consume 200 mg of caffeine, it can take 3 to 5 hours for half of it to leave your body, and 18 to 24 hours to get rid of the rest of it. This leads to a vicious cycle; you have trouble falling asleep, which leads you to wake up even more tired and needing caffeine again.

Not All Caffeinated Drinks Are Created Alike

Espresso: 30 to 50 mg of caffeine per shot

97 percent decaf coffee: 3 to 6 mg per 6 ounces

Drip-brewed coffee: 75 to 200 mg per 6 ounces

Red Bull: 80 mg per 8.5 ounces

Jolt Endurance shot: 200 mg per 2 ounces

Caffeinated sodas: 20 to 26 mg per 6 ounces

Black tea: 40 to 60 mg per 8 ounces

Dark chocolate: 20 mg per ounce

Hot chocolate: 10 to 15 mg per 6 ounces

The Nurses' Health Study did point to one particular caffeine-related danger. Intake of caffeinated soft drinks was associated with a higher risk of ovulatory infertility among women who drank two or more per day. Similar associations were also observed for non-caffeinated, sugared soft drinks, so I would recommend avoiding sodas, which are really an empty, high-glycemic-load form of calories. Diet sodas are not the answer, either; the chemical sweeteners in diet sodas may pose health risks, and paradoxically, drinking diet soda has been shown to increase waist circumferences.

Seafood and Fertility

As I mentioned, it's crucial to consume omega-3s while attempting to conceive. Omega-3s are important for both your baby's neural development and for preventing postpartum depression. Most Americans are sorely deficient in omega-3s, which is why normalizing your levels before conception is so essential. However, since the FDA/EPA put out their fish advisory in 2004, warning pregnant women to eat no more than 12 ounces per week of seafood, many women have responded by not eating any fish whatsoever. Data from the National Health and Nutrition Examination

71

Survey (NHANES) shows that 90 percent of women are consuming less than the FDA-recommended amount of fish.

Several recent studies have looked into the value of eating fish during pregnancy. An important one is the Avon Longitudinal Study of Parents and Children, which began in 1991 in Bristol, England, and is following children throughout their lives to determine the impact of environment, nutrition, and other factors on their development. Led by Dr. Joseph Hibbeln of the United States National Institutes of Health, the study tracked the eating habits of 11,875 pregnant women.

Thus far, the study has shown that the children of women who ate less than 340 grams (two or three servings) of seafood per week while pregnant had significantly lower IQs. Children whose moms ate no seafood were 48 percent more likely to have a low verbal IQ. In addition, women who ate three or more servings of seafood per week had children with better neurological function. The researchers concluded that women who avoid seafood during pregnancy may actually harm their infants by depriving them of nutrients required for fetal brain development.

Another study, of 643 children in the Seychelles Islands, began in 2003 and followed pregnant women who were eating an average of twelve fish meals per week. The study reported that there was no evidence of risk to the children from mercury consumed with the fish. It was theorized that since fish contain omega-3s, iodine, iron, and choline, the benefits from those nutrients countered the potential risk of mercury.

Yet despite all this new evidence about eating fish, the FDA/EPA still recommends consuming less than 340 grams per week during pregnancy.

From my perspective, we often fall into the trap of thinking that if a little is good, more is better. This leads women to go off fish completely when trying to conceive and when pregnant. The EPA warning about not eating fish high in mercury, such as shark, king mackerel, swordfish, or tilefish, is good advice, since big predator fish bioaccumulate, thus concentrating more mercury in their flesh as they feed on smaller fish. However, deciding not to eat fish at all is an inappropriate response, as these studies show.

Sushi, a favorite food for many, is also a major culprit when it comes to mercury exposure; the National Resources Defense Council has compiled a list of fish used in sushi and its levels of mercury. Many of the most popular types of sushi contain high levels of mercury and should be completely avoided. Entirely avoid *kajiki* (swordfish), *saba* (mackerel), shark, and tilefish. In addition, don't eat more than three 6-ounce servings per month of *ahi, buri, hamachi, inada,* or *kanpachi* (yellowfin tuna); *katsuo* (bonito); *meji* (young bigeye, bluefin, or yellowfin tuna); *maguro* (bigeye or bluefin tuna); *makjiki* (blue marlin); *masu* (trout); *shiro* (albacore); or *toro* (yellowfin or bigeye). Below is a full list of sushi recommendations.

Sushi Recommendations for Those Trying to Conceive
(chart obtained from the Natural Resources Defense Council [NRDC]; data obtained by the FDA and the EPA)

The NRDC has compiled a list of fish used in sushi and their levels of mercury. Many of the main sushi-type fish contain high levels of mercury and should be completely avoided. If you have further questions regarding sushi, you should talk with your healthcare provider to get a recommendation.

HIGHEST MERCURY
Avoid the following:
Kajiki (swordfish)
Saba (mackerel)
Shark
Tilefish

HIGH MERCURY
Eat no more than three 6-ounce servings per month.
Ahi (yellowfin tuna)
Buri (adult yellowtail)

Hamachi (young yellowtail)

Inada (very young yellowtail)

Kanpachi (very young yellowtail)

Katsuo (bonito)

Maguro (bigeye, bluefin, or yellowfin tuna)

Makjiki (blue marlin)

Masu (trout)

Meji (young bigeye, bluefin, or yellowfin tuna)

Shiro (albacore tuna)

Toro (bigeye, bluefin, or yellowfin tuna)

LOWER MERCURY

Eat no more than six 6-ounce servings per month.

Kani (crab)

Seigo (young sea bass)

Suzuki (sea bass)

LOWEST MERCURY

Enjoy two 6-ounce servings per week.

Aji (horse mackerel)

Akagai (ark shell)

Anago (conger eel)

Aoyagi (round clam)

Awabi (abalone)

Ayu (sweetfish)

Ebi (shrimp)

Hamaguri (clam)

Hamo (pike conger, sea eel)

Hatahata (sandfish)

Himo (ark shell)

Hokkigai (surf clam)

Hotategai (scallop)

Ika (squid)

Ikura (salmon roe)

Kaibashira (shellfish)

Karei (flatfish)

Kohada (gizzard shad)

Masago (smelt egg)

Mirugai (surf clam)

Nori-tama (egg)

Sake (salmon)

Sawara (Spanish mackerel)

Sayori (halfbeak)

Shako (mantis shrimp)

Tai (sea bream)

Tairagai (razor-shell clam)

Tako (octopus)

Tamago (egg)

Tobikko (flying fish egg)

Torigai (cockle)

Tsubugai (shellfish)

Unagi (freshwater eel)

Uni (sea urchin roe)

Many women have asked me if they should be tested for mercury levels when they begin to think about getting pregnant. Testing for mercury is expensive and time-consuming, as it involves twenty-four-hour urine monitoring. That said, women who have been consuming a lot of fish with high mercury levels, such as tuna, might consider testing before preparing to conceive.

Other Sources of Omega-3

Some people believe that flaxseed or flaxseed oil is equivalent to fish, and take it for its omega-3 content. I often recommend ground flax as a wonderful addition to the diet. In addition to omega-3, it contains fiber (which most of us don't get enough of) and lignans (which reduce the risk of breast and prostate cancer). Unfortunately, flax contains the shorter chain alpha-linolenic acid (ALA), which does not convert substantially into the longer chain fatty acids—EPA (eicosapentaenoic acid) and DHA (docosahexaenoic acid)—that are essential to our overall health. This is also true for other plant omega-3 sources such as hemp seed, walnuts, and purslane; all are healthy forms of ALA, but since women convert only 21 percent of it to EPA and 9 percent to DHA, they are not sufficient sources of omega-3. (Men convert even less ALA to the longer-chain fatty acids, averaging 8 percent to EPA and 0 to 4 percent to DHA.)

What I do recommend are omega-3–enriched eggs, which have three to six times the omega-3s of regular eggs, and are worth the extra cost. Omega-3 eggs are laid by chickens that have been fed either flax or algae. One omega-3–enriched egg has up to 500 mg of ALA and 150 mg of DHA per yolk, depending on the egg's size and what the chickens were fed; be sure to check the carton label to determine how much omega-3 fats are in the eggs. But don't be fooled by total omega-3: it's the DHA and EPA content that is most important.

Eggs can be of value for another reason. While we all want our cholesterol to be low, when a woman has very low cholesterol, she may not manufacture adequate amounts of sex hormones (since cholesterol is the precursor for production of these hormones). Therefore, adding eggs can be a therapeutic option for women with low cholesterol.

I believe it's important to buy only organic eggs, preferably those with extra omega-3. Shockingly, arsenic has been used as a growth promoter and an antimicrobial in conventional chicken farms, so if the eggs aren't organic, you may well be ingesting arsenic. In July 2010, the *Salt Lake Tribune* reported that two children who had been eating eight to ten eggs per week from their families' backyard chicken coops had alarmingly high levels of arsenic in their bodies. It turned out that the families weren't using organic feed; the feed contained arsenic additives, which wound up in the children.

Ideally, all of our omega-3 needs are met by fish and eggs. However, given the sad environmental challenges facing our oceans, and the need to be selective about fish choices, I also recommend supplementing with fish oil. We can buy fish oil without any mercury (since products are molecularly distilled, which removes the mercury, lead, and PCBs), rendering fish oil safer than fish. In Chapter 4, "Supplements," I will review doses and what to look for on the label.

Vitamin D

Fish not only provides us omega-3s but also is one of the few food sources of vitamin D; 75 grams of cooked salmon contains 225 IU of vitamin D, and 75 grams of tuna, 41 IU of vitamin D. There is some evidence that you cannot get pregnant if you don't have enough vitamin D in your body. I recommend that all women have a blood test to assess their vitamin D levels, and then decide whether to supplement.

Vitamin D is called the sunshine vitamin because it is formed in our skin through sun exposure. Sunscreen effectively blocks this (an unintended consequence of a serious nature), and those who live in latitudes north of Atlanta cannot form vitamin D in the winter months. Foods fortified with vitamin D can help. One cup of milk has 100 IU of vitamin D; a cup of soy milk has 80 IU; a cup of fortified orange juice contains 90 IU. I'll have more to say about vitamin D in "Supplements."

Alcohol and Fertility

Alcohol intake is often a sensitive topic. More than sixteen studies have looked at the association between alcohol and fertility; considering the mixed results, I don't think you have to completely abstain from what might be your favorite beverage when trying to get pregnant. In the Nurses' Health Study, for example, there was no association between one alcoholic drink per day and ovulatory infertility.

Having said that, studies show that most women rapidly stop drinking alcohol once they know they are pregnant. Since you don't know when you are going to

77

conceive, and since the early stage of pregnancy is so important for your baby's brain development, I'd suggest limiting yourself to no more than one drink per day. (See page 46 for definition of "one drink.")

Mindful Eating

A final consideration for the woman who wants to conceive is eating mindfully. Mindfulness is the quality of paying attention to and being aware of the present moment. Consider the difference between what it means to nourish yourself and to eat on the run. In modern-day life, we often are so rushed for time that we eat in the car, at our desks, or even while standing in the kitchen watching the news on TV. Wolfing down food in this way, we rarely focus on what we are putting into our bodies. This lack of attention can cause us to miss the chance to savor each bite, as well as lead to overeating and to eating foods that aren't good for us.

Mindful eating is the opposite. In *Coming to Our Senses,* mindfulness teacher Jon Kabat-Zinn says, "When we taste with attention, even the simplest foods provide a universe of sensory experience, awakening us to them."

Kabat-Zinn uses a meditation called the Raisin Exercise, which promotes mindful eating. I have excerpted it below (with permission from Random House) from his book *Full Catastrophe Living.* Do the exercise alone or with a family member or friend, and be prepared to be shocked at how little you have noticed about the full flavor of a raisin. For a special treat, use a chocolate-covered (organic) strawberry instead.

> First we bring our attention to seeing the raisin, observing it carefully as if we had never seen one before. We feel its texture between our fingers and notice its colors and surfaces. We are also aware of any thoughts we might be having about raisins or food in general. We note any thoughts and feelings of liking or disliking raisins. . . . We then smell it for a while and finally, with awareness, we bring it to our lips, being aware of the arm moving the hand to position it correctly and of salivating as the mind and body anticipate eating. The process continues as we take it into our mouth and chew it

slowly, experiencing the actual taste of one raisin. And when we feel ready to swallow, we watch the impulse to swallow as it comes up, so that even that is experienced consciously. We even imagine, or "sense," that now our bodies are one raisin heavier.

Use the lesson of the Raisin Exercise to slow down your eating and to become more conscious and mindful of the way in which you nourish your body. Another way to practice more mindful eating is to turn off the television, radio, and your cell phone while you eat. You not only avoid ads for snack foods, for example, but also become more aware of each bite as you put it into your mouth.

Mindful eating serves another purpose: it makes us generally more mindful. As we consider bearing children, we think about what we wish to model for them and the parents we hope to be. Children pay careful attention to what their parents do, as opposed to what they say. Getting into the habit of eating healthfully and mindfully now, while you're trying to get pregnant, not only strengthens your health and that of your baby, but also provides an example worth following for your child.

CHAPTER FOUR

SUPPLEMENTS

I n 1982, as a medical student, I was taught that people don't need to take vitamins if they eat a healthy diet. Believe it or not, the debate about the value of multivitamins continues today. In any event, the point may be moot, as too many Americans neither eat a healthy diet nor get the recommended daily allowances of nutrients. The Centers for Disease Control (CDC) data shows that 75 percent of the U.S. population is not meeting the daily requirement for folate; 34 percent do not get enough iron; 42 percent don't get enough zinc; and 73 percent are deficient in calcium. This is because our Western, largely processed-food diet is low in vegetables and fruits, where many of the nutrients we need reside. As a nation, we have become overweight and undernourished. Ideally, I ask my patients to address this by eating a healthful diet as outlined in the previous chapter. To be totally explicit: supplements *cannot* replace the value of a nutritious diet. Still, there are times, conception being one of the most critical, when supplements—and especially multivitamins—are advisable.

The 2011 National Health and Nutrition Examination Survey (NHANES) revealed that supplements are widely used by Americans over the age of twenty, with multivitamins being the most common of all; 53 percent of Americans took them in 2003–2006. However, only 34 percent of women ages twenty to thirty-nine get the recommended amount of supplemental folic acid. This poses a significant problem when it comes to conception. In this chapter, I will tell you why multivitamins and folic acid are so important. I will also point you to other recommended supplements that can help you conceive, but first I want to explain the state of the dietary supplement industry in America.

Regulation of Supplements

In 1994, the government was going to drastically limit the types and content of dietary supplements in the marketplace. In response, concerned Americans began the largest letter-writing campaign to Congress since the Vietnam War. As a result of public pressure, Congress passed the Dietary Supplement Health and Education Act (DSHEA), which defined dietary supplements as vitamins, minerals, herbs and botanicals, amino acids, and other dietary substances such as enzymes. The good news was that DSHEA left consumers with wide access to supplements. The downside is that dietary supplements are less stringently regulated than pharmaceuticals. It is the companies themselves that are responsible for ensuring that high-quality products go on the market; supplements are investigated by the FDA only if there are complaints about them. DSHEA allows only structure function claims; for example, a company can't say that cranberry helps prevent urinary tract infections, only that it helps support bladder health. The overall effect of DSHEA is that consumers have to do a lot of work to figure out which products to take, and whether they are of high quality.

Thirteen years after DSHEA was passed, in 2007, regulations were implemented that require all companies to ensure that their products are made consistently in a high-quality manner, are accurately labeled, and are free from impurities. In addition—and this may seem surprising—each product must contain what the label says it does, nothing more (e.g., adulterants) and nothing less. The manufacturer must employ quality-control procedures, test the raw ingredients as well as the finished product, and have a way to handle consumer complaints. These new rules have improved the quality of many of the dietary supplements available on the market today.

Herbs and botanicals pose additional challenges. As a consumer, you need to be cognizant of the part of the plant that is said to have medicinal properties, as it could be the leaf, root, or flower. Herbalists remind us that the potency of herbs can vary from year to year, depending on the amount of rainfall, the quality of the soil, and when the plant was harvested. Other influences include how the plant was dried, stored, and prepared. This gives you some sense of the complexity of preparing herbal medicines.

One way to distinguish higher quality supplements is to buy from companies that avail themselves of third-party testing of their products. The U.S. Pharmacopeial Convention (USP), the National Sanitation Foundation (NSF), and the National Products Association (NPA) set standards and provide inspections. Companies that pass such inspections can put a USP or NSF label on their products, which can help you to select wisely. Another independent testing group, Consumer Labs, has a site (www.consumerlabs.com), which you can currently join for $33 per year, that offers another way to check on product quality. Since supplements are costly, joining the site may well be a money-saving strategy over the course of a year.

Should You Take a Multivitamin?

Men and women preparing for pregnancy are wise to take multivitamins. Exposure to oxidative stress from diet, stress, exercise, and environmental chemicals creates reactive oxygen molecules. In women, these reactive oxygen species (ROS) can affect how well the egg matures, how easily it is fertilized, and how well the embryo develops. ROS may also contribute to the age-related decline in fertility, and oxidative stress also has a significant impact on spermatogenesis; taking a multi can enhance a man's fertility.

Scientific studies suggest that there are four major reasons to take a multivitamin. First, we know from the Nurses' Health Study that taking multis help a woman get pregnant. Women in the study who took multis had a third lower risk of developing

83

ovulatory infertility, compared with nonusers. The researchers estimated that 20 percent of all ovulatory infertility cases could be avoided if women took a multi at least three times per week. Another study found that women who took multis were more fertile than those who did not. This simple intervention can have a marked effect on fertility.

Second, multivitamins help prevent birth defects. A Canadian meta-analysis that looked at forty-one studies evaluating the use of multivitamins with folic acid before conception and through the third trimester found that taking a multivitamin provided protection against neural tube defects, cardiovascular defects, limb defects, cleft palate, and urinary-tract anomalies. The degree of protection ranged from 25 percent to over 50 percent for these various birth defects.

Third, taking a multivitamin helps to prevent miscarriage. A 2007 research trial showed that vitamin supplementation in the first trimester was associated with a 50 percent reduced risk of miscarriage. Finally, women who take multis during pregnancy have fewer children with pediatric cancer. Cancer is the second leading cause of death in children; recent studies show that maternal prenatal multivitamin consumption reduces the risk of pediatric cancer later in life.

Four Reasons to Take a Multivitamin

1. Taking a multi may help you to conceive.
2. Taking a multi reduces the risk of birth defects in your baby.
3. Taking a multi lowers the risk of miscarriage.
4. Taking a multi reduces the risk of pediatric cancer in your child.

Preliminary research provides a fifth reason to take multivitamins before you become pregnant. Two studies that came out in 2011 suggest that preconceptual vitamins may reduce the risk of autism and other learning disabilities. The CHARGE (Childhood Autism Risks from Genetics and Environment) study was a case control study carried out in Northern California. It assessed the impact of maternal prenatal vitamin consumption in 269 children with typical development, as compared to 276 children with autism. The mothers who began taking prenatal vitamins in the three months prior to and up to one month into pregnancy had a 38 percent reduced risk of autism in their children, as compared to those mothers who did not begin multivtamins until later in pregnancy. A Norwegian study looked at the impact of maternal supplementation from four weeks prior to eight weeks after conception in almost 39,000 children. (Of note, Norway does not fortify food with folic acid, which increases the contrast between women who do and don't take supplements.) They found that mothers who took folic acid alone or folic acid plus other vitamins had a 45 percent lower risk of having children with severe language delays at age three.

I recommend to my patients that they take a multivitamin every single day. Begin taking them the moment you start thinking about conceiving—and because pregnancies are not always planned, it is wise for all young adults to take them. It may well help you to conceive, and it will ensure that when you do conceive, you lower the risk of birth defects and miscarriage. Some find that multivitamins are difficult to swallow, or that they cause nausea. First thing in the morning, on an empty stomach, can be especially difficult. Instead, take them with the largest meal of the day (usually lunch or dinner). I find swallowing my supplements between bites of food helps. If you suffer "fish burps," freeze your omega-3 and take it with dinner.

While prenatal vitamins are often recommended, check the ingredient list against the list below with care. Multis can have twenty-five or more different ingredients. This helps ensure that you get the variety of vitamins and trace minerals that impact fertility, and mitigate gaps in the diet. Prenatal vitamins are designed to have the extra folic acid needed when you are seeking to conceive. Iron and iodine are usually added; however, amounts vary. Some have added DHA (one of the long-chain omegas) but fewer have EPA. Most prenatal vitamins will not contain all the omega-3, vitamin D, and calcium recommended—so you will likely need more than one pill. Some recommended amounts of vitamins and minerals vary from the preconception period to pregnancy to after your baby is born. Suffice it to say that not all multivitamins are created alike! Be sure that yours includes vitamins A, C, and D, folic acid, and the minerals calcium, iron, and iodine.

What to Look for in Your Multivitamin

1. Check the vitamin A first for a maximum of 2,500 IU of vitamin A as vitamin A palmitate, vitamin A acetate, or retinol palmitate. Up to 15,000 IU of beta-carotene is allowable. It's fine if it reads vitamin A 100 percent as beta-carotene.

2. Be sure it contains iron 18 mg (most men should not take supplemental iron).

3. Iodine should be 150 mcg.

4. Folic acid should be 400 or more mcg (it's okay to have up to 1,000 mcg or 1 gm).

5. DHA may not be in it at all. If it is, look for a dose of 300 mg or more. Ideally EPA is in your vitamin as well. Most likely you will need to take fish oil capsule(s) in addition to your multi. Look for a molecularly distilled omega-3 with 300 to 400 mg of DHA and 500 mg of EPA, and take it with your largest meal of the day.

6. Vitamin D—you will want at least 1,000 IU per day (or more if your lab work shows you to be deficient). Most multis won't have this much and you will need to add an additional supplement. Vitamin D_3 (cholecalciferol) is recommended but vegan products will likely have vitamin D_2 (ergocalciferol) and this is okay, too.

7. Vitamin E—do not buy a multi with dl alpha tocopherol—it's the synthetic form, and a sign of a poor product. If the label reads *d-alpha tocopherol*, that is okay; better yet are 200 to 400 IU of mixed tocopherols and tocotrienols.

8. Vitamin B_{12} (cyanocobalamin): 2.4 mcg.
9. Other vitamins: a multi will likely contain vitamins C and B (there is a whole family of B vitamins—B_1, also called thiamine; B_2, also called riboflavin; B_6, also called pyridoxine Hcl; B_3, which is Niacin or Niacinamide; B_{12} [cyanocobalamin]; B_7 [Biotin]; and B_5 [pantothenic acid]).
10. Trace minerals: a multi should also contain small amounts of copper, zinc, magnesium, potassium, and calcium. (You will likely need to supplement with some additional calcium.)

Vitamin A

Vitamin A is important for the fetus's developing vision and immune function. Dietary sources of vitamin A include leafy vegetables, carrots, sweet potatoes, egg yolks, whole milk, and liver. When animal products are the source of vitamin A, it is often referred to as preformed vitamin A. Absorbed in the form of retinol, this preformed A is easily assimilated into our bodies. Fruits and vegetables are the primary source of the pro-vitamin A carotenoids such as beta-carotene. There are more than five hundred such carotenoids, and they provide many health benefits. However, only about 10 percent of the carotenoids are converted into active forms of vitamin A in our bodies.

Vitamin A is critical to our health, but it has a narrow therapeutic window. Since many foods are fortified with vitamin A, it is possible to get too much. An excess of vitamin A while pregnant increases the risk of birth defects. On your multivitamin ingredient label, first check for vitamin A. Preformed vitamin A will be listed as vitamin A palmitate, vitamin A acetate, or retinol palmitate. You want a maximum of 2,500 IUs per day. If your label reads vitamin A as beta-carotene, there can be as much as 15,000 IU and still be safe. (Once you get pregnant, taking 5,000 IU beta-carotene is considered safe. We simply don't know about higher doses.)

Folic Acid

Another critical ingredient in your multi is folic acid, which is required for the synthesis of DNA and cell division. DNA is essential to reproduction and impacts the quality of the oocyte. The word *folate* comes from the same root as foliage. Not surprisingly, green leafy vegetables are a rich source of folate in the diet. Folate is also found in legumes, citrus fruits and juices, and breads and cereals made with folic acid–enriched flour. (I have suggested, however, that you avoid these high-glycemic-load foods made from flour.) Despite food fortification, 90 percent of women do not get sufficient folic acid from the diet, and only 20 percent of women are taking a multi with folic acid.

Multiple professional organizations, including the U.S. Public Health Service, the American Academy of Pediatrics, the American Academy of Family Medicine, and the American College of Obstetricians and Gynecologists, recommend that *all* women of childbearing age take 400 mcg of folic acid daily, because it helps prevent neural tube defects.

In the United States, half of all pregnancies are unplanned. Yet to prevent neural defects, folic acid has to be on board from the earliest stages of development; beginning to supplement at eight to twelve weeks of pregnancy is simply too late. There is some evidence that folate increases the likelihood of twin births, but the balance weighs heavily in favor of supplementation.

Iodine

One of the essential trace minerals that we rarely think about is iodine. Iodine performs one key role in the body: it is used to make thyroid hormone. Food sources of iodine include milk, egg yolks, saltwater fish, garlic, sesame seeds, asparagus, spinach, lima beans, soybeans, mushrooms, seaweed, dulse, and kelp. In the early 1900s, many Americans had goiter, an enlarged, overworked thyroid, resulting from iodine deficiency. Scientists and public health officials worked with salt manufacturers to add iodine to salt. In most of the developed world, table salt has now been supplemented with iodine. Salt was selected because it is easy to iodize and inexpensive; its intake is uniform across socioeconomic strata, and doesn't vary from season to season.

Yet iodine deficiency increased in the United States from 1 percent of pregnant women in 1974 to 7 percent in 1994. Processed food, although heavily salted, is not made with iodized salt. Sea salt, which is growing in popularity, naturally contains some iodine, but is not a reliable source. Public health messages have encouraged people to cut back on their salt intake. And finally, in areas where the groundwater has been contaminated with perchlorate, our ability to take iodine up into the thyroid is compromised. A borderline low iodine level (< 100 mcg/d) plus perchlorate spells clinical hypothyroidism.

The World Health Organization estimates that two billion people in the world are iodine-deficient, and that iodine is the single most common cause of preventable mental retardation and brain damage in the world. Iodine deficiency also causes miscarriage and stillbirths.

A urine iodine test can assess your level. If it comes back low, be sure there is iodine in your multivitamin and that you are taking it every day; in addition, use more iodized salt. The recommended daily iodine allowance is 150 mcg during preconception, and 200 mcg while pregnant or breast-feeding.

Omega-3

As I mentioned earlier, omega-3 is especially important when preparing to conceive and when pregnant. There are two long-chain omega-3 fatty acids that you want to look for in an omega-3 supplement: DHA (docosahexaenoic acid) and EPA (eicosopentaenoic acid). Alpha-linolenic acid may also show up on the label, as may omega 3–6–9. It is really DHA and EPA that need supplementation.

DHA is so important to fetal brain development that a pregnant woman's body will transfer all it can across the placenta to nourish the baby even at the expense of the mother becoming depleted. EPA is needed to prevent postpartum depression. While the consumption of fish, as opposed to fish-oil supplements, is best studied for these effects, as well as to prevent preterm labor, widespread fish contamination makes these supplements an important option. Fish-oil supplements are molecularly distilled (look for this on the label), which effectively removes the heavy metal and PCB contaminants present in many fish.

A Canadian survey of 176 pregnant women revealed that while 90 percent were taking multivitamins, none were taking the vitamins with omega-3, and only 11 percent were taking separate omega-3 supplements. In randomized trials using a DHA supplement versus a placebo, the supplement improved infants' visual acuity and growth as well as helped prevent maternal depression. Omega-3 supplementation has also been shown to extend gestation and increase birth weight. While more studies need to be done to determine the ideal dose, we do know that it is safe to take omega-3 supplements during pregnancy. Look for a molecularly distilled omega-3 with 300 to 400 mg of DHA and 500 to 600 mg of EPA, and take it with your largest meal of the day.

Iron

Iron deficiency is common in women; the National Health and Nutrition Examination Survey study showed that 9 to 16 percent of women between the ages of twelve and forty-nine are iron deficient, and fully 40 percent of women have virtually no iron reserves in their bodies. Iron reserves are reduced by blood loss during menstruation and childbirth; in addition, many women's diets don't contain much iron. Only 20 percent of fertile women have good iron reserves of 500 mg.

If a woman has iron deficiency anemia before conception, it can impair how the placenta develops early in pregnancy. Reduced infant growth and an increased risk of poorer pregnancy outcomes may result, so restoring iron levels prior to conception is recommended. And do keep in mind that vitamin C can enhance iron absorption.

In the Nurses' Health Study, women who took iron supplements had a 40 percent lower risk of ovulatory infertility than those who didn't take them. The CDC recommends 18 mg of iron per day for preconception, and 27 mg per day for a pregnant woman. Many women avoid taking iron supplements due to their constipating effects; using food-based iron supplements or iron bisglycinate can reduce this side effect.

Vitamin D

Many women have low vitamin D levels. This is because many of us live in northern latitudes where we can't make vitamin D in the winter months. Or we follow our dermatologists' recommendations and slather on sunscreen, which, while protecting us from skin cancer, also blocks our ability to form vitamin D in our skin. There is evidence in animal studies and some from human trials that fertility is impaired if the mother has a low vitamin D level. She will have a harder time getting pregnant, and once pregnant, she will have an increased risk of preeclampsia and gestational diabetes. Thus, I recommend that women have their vitamin D levels checked.

The Institute of Medicine considers doses of up to 4,000 IUs of vitamin D per day to be safe. Many multivitamins contain only 200 IUs; this dose is unlikely to be adequate in someone who is seriously depleted. In fact, when someone is very deficient, doctors often prescribe a dose of 25,000 IUs of vitamin D2 per week. Alternatively, some doctors suggest a daily 5,000 IU, over-the-counter dose of vitamin D3 for a total of 35,000 IU per week. By having your level checked, your physician can more accurately prescribe the right dose for you.

Calcium

Calcium is also important during pregnancy and breast-feeding; we need 1,000 to 1,300 mg per day. In addition to dairy foods, calcium is found in sardines, salmon, figs, broccoli, and almonds, to name a few sources; however, most people don't get enough calcium in their diets alone. When supplementing, it is best to split your dose, as we can't absorb more than about 500 mg of calcium at any one time. Of note, a recent study showed that lead levels declined in women who took 600 mg of calcium twice a day. This is an intriguing method to deal with a serious environmental concern.

B_{12}

Another vitamin to consider taking is B_{12}. If you are a vegan or strict vegetarian, have been taking a proton pump inhibitor or other acid blocker, or have been on oral contraceptives for a number of years, you are at higher risk for having a low B_{12} level. Metformin, often prescribed for PCOS, also depletes B_{12} levels. Among its varied roles, vitamin B_{12} is required for DNA synthesis; low levels raise the risks of repeated miscarriage and birth defects. Vitamin B_{12} is naturally found in animal products, including fish, meat, poultry, eggs, milk, and milk products; it is also in fortified cereals. Recommended dietary allowances are 2.4 mcg preconception and 2.6 mcg when pregnant. A supplement with 1,000 mcg of oral B_{12} leads you to absorb about 20 mcg, which is enough to correct B_{12} deficiency in about eight weeks. Oral B_{12} supplementation works for most people.

Additional Supplements to Consider

Probiotics

Normally the human digestive tract has four hundred different types of probiotic bacteria, which inhibit the growth of harmful bacteria and promote a healthy digestive system. Yet antibiotics, which most of us have taken at some point, reduce the diverse microflora of the gut. We now know that microbes have important effects on our immune system, and that we actually have more bacterial DNA in our bodies than human DNA. The fetal programming hypothesis holds that exposure to microbes before conception, during pregnancy, and in the neonatal period has profound effects on the baby's developing immune system. For these reasons, it may be worth taking a probiotic before you conceive. Kevin Coughlin, MD, a family physician, acupuncturist, and graduate of our fellowship, also recommends probiotics to lower vaginal inflammation and to increase the absorption of nutrients. A probiotic supplement is one strategy that I recommend; another is to eat probiotic-rich Greek yogurt several times a week.

Antioxidants

Antioxidants accumulate in the ovaries and help preovulatory follicles grow and develop in response to hormone stimulation. One study that supports the use of vitamin C (an antioxidant vitamin) followed 150 women who had luteal phase defects. The experimental group took 750 mg of vitamin C per day; after six months, there was a 25 percent rate of pregnancy, compared to 11 percent in the control group. Progesterone levels were significantly elevated in the vitamin C–treated group, with a 52 percent increase versus 22 percent in the placebo group. Taking supplemental vitamin C is a very simple intervention that may help women with luteal phase defects. Another study, which treated women undergoing IVF with 500 mg of vitamin C during their follicular phases, found a trend toward higher pregnancy rates among the group.

Fertility Blend

Vitamin C is one of the components of a combined antioxidant product called Fertility Blend, which is a proprietary mixture of chasteberry, green tea extract, L-arginine, vitamin C, B$_6$, B$_{12}$, folate, iron, magnesium, zinc, and selenium. Two studies were done on this product. The pilot study involved thirty women ages twenty-four to forty-six who hadn't been able to conceive after six to thirty-six months. After taking Fertility Blend for five months, 33 percent of the women were pregnant, versus zero with a placebo.

In 2006, the study was repeated with ninety-three women ages twenty-four to forty-two who had been unable to conceive for six to thirty-six months. After three months, Fertility Blend showed a trend toward increasing mid-luteal progesterone levels. For the women who had low progesterone to begin with, the increase was highly significant. Pregnancy rates improved, as well: 26 percent versus 10 percent for the placebo. Dr. Lynn Westphal, the Stanford reproductive endocrinologist who conducted the studies, considers Fertility Blend a useful supplement especially for women with irregular cycles. The company has also produced a Fertility Blend for men, although there are no published studies available for this product.

N-acetyl Cysteine

Another antioxidant supplement to consider is N-acetyl cysteine, which has been used in conjunction with the ovulation-inducing medication Clomid. One trial studied a dose of 1,200 mg versus a placebo, combined with 100 mg of Clomid. It showed increased ovulation and pregnancy rates in women ages eighteen to thirty-nine who had Clomid-resistant PCOS. The addition of N-acetyl cysteine was more effective than the placebo. Women who took the combination ovulated 49 percent of the time, versus 1 percent with Clomid alone; pregnancy rate was 21 percent, compared with zero in Clomid alone. While not all studies were positive, this is another supplement to consider with or without the Clomid, since it's quite safe.

Herbs and Supplements

Herbs are used quite differently by different practitioners. A physician can prescribe a carefully standardized herbal product, knowing the exact amounts of each part of the plant that has been included and the exact dose. Essentially this is similar to prescribing a high-grade pharmaceutical herb in place of a medicine. At the other end of the spectrum is the traditional herbalist perspective. Herbs are said to nourish and tonify the uterus, to relax the nervous system, and to establish and balance the hormonal system. Dr. Maggie Ney, a naturopathic physician with whom I spoke about the use of herbs, explains that terms like *adaptogen, nourishing,* and *tonifying* speak to both the energetic and pharmacological properties of the herb, which are believed to support a particular organ's strength and vitality. Dr. Tieraona Low Dog, director of the Fellowship at the Arizona Center for Integrative Medicine, and past chairwoman of the U.S. Pharmacopeia Subcommittee on Dietary Supplements, is one of the world's leading experts on botanicals. She is passionate about women's health, and in 2010 coedited with me the Oxford University Press text *Integrative Women's Health*. Dr. Low Dog believes that herbal medicine has a place in supporting fertility, and that herbs can be a midway point between drugs and surgical intervention.

There is a long traditional history of herbal remedies for all aspects of reproductive health, from menstruation through conception and pregnancy. Unfortunately, there are not many studies that show conclusively how effective herbs can be. For our purposes, I will focus on some of the herbs that have been best studied, and briefly mention other common herbal remedies.

If you are drawn to herbal medicine, it might be good to work with an experienced herbalist or naturopathic physician. To find an herbalist, check with the American Herbalist Guild, which registers professional medical herbalists who have completed a rigorous review process. An herb that may help balance your menstrual cycle might not be the right thing to use once you are pregnant. Exercise caution, as some herbs are emmenagogues; they can increase the risk of miscarriage or abortion.

Vitex agnus-castus

Vitex agnus-castus, or chasteberry, is one of the best-studied herbs. Derived from a berry-bearing shrub, its medicinal properties are partly related to its essential oils. *Vitex* has been shown to reduce levels of follicle-stimulating hormone and increase luteinizing hormone, thereby reducing estrogen and increasing progesterone. At higher amounts, it can inhibit prolactin levels. Thus it can be especially helpful in women who have luteal phase disorders.

    Vitex has been studied as one component of Fertility Blend, discussed above; it has also been researched for fertility on its own in two European trials. The first showed that the pregnancy rate in ninety-six women who received *Vitex* was 23 percent, twice as high as that in the placebo group. The highest success was seen in women who had luteal insufficiency. A smaller trial, of fifty-two women, looked at the effect of *Vitex* on luteal phase defect. Prolactin was reduced, progesterone concentration improved, beta estradiol increased, and two women conceived (versus none in the placebo group). *Vitex* is definitely an herb to consider if you have a luteal phase defect. Dr. Low Dog has also found *Vitex* to be effective for women who have repeated miscarriages in the eighth or tenth week, possibly due to its favorable effects on progesterone.

Shatavari Root

Shatavari root, or *Asparagus racemosus,* is commonly used in Ayurvedic medicine; the name *shatavari* translates to "she who possesses one hundred husbands." Shatavari is a female reproductive nutritive tonic that has been used for fertility in India for more than a thousand years. An adaptogenic herb, it has many beneficial properties: it is an antioxidant, is antitumor and antibacterial, increases insulin secretion, decreases stomach acid and prevents stress ulcers, and stimulates the immune response. Damiana, or *Turnera aphrodisiaca,* is the Western hemisphere equivalent to shatavari. Note the reference to its aphrodisiac reputation in the Latin name. In Mexico, one can find damiana liqueurs in bottles designed to look like a voluptuous woman. Traditionally, when women married, they were given damiana for the first thirty days after their ceremonies to enhance the chance of getting pregnant.

    Dr. Low Dog shared with me her tasty recipe for shatavari. Take an ounce of shatavari root; put it into 4 cups of soy, rice, almond, or regular milk; and cook it in a small lidded saucepan over a very low flame for 20 minutes. Strain the liquid and return it to the heat; add ¼ teaspoon cardamom and 1 to 2 tablespoons honey or raw sugar. Gently heat until mixed, then cool, cover, and put into the fridge. Drink one cup per day.

Additional Herbs Commonly Suggested for Fertility

Below are some additional herbs that are commonly suggested for fertility. Most have not been tested for safety in pregnancy. One way to approach their use is to take them in the first half of the menstrual cycle and stop at ovulation.

Red clover flower (*Trifolium pratense*) is said to have a high vitamin and protein content. It also contains calcium and magnesium, and is a rich source of trace minerals. Red clover helps alkalinize the body, which may help balance the pH in the vagina in favor of conception. You can infuse an ounce of red clover with a little bit of peppermint in a quart of water for four hours, and drink it several times a day. Red clover tea is quite safe, but you should probably avoid taking the extracts; these concentrated products are high in isoflavones, and their safety in pregnancy is uncertain.

Red raspberry leaf (*Rubus idaeus*) is a uterine tonic. A rich source of calcium, it is often combined with red clover flower, and is said to help prevent miscarriage and increase fertility in men and women. Red raspberry leaf has been studied in pregnant women, and there are no known adverse effects. Steep ½ ounce red clover blossoms and ½ ounce red raspberry leaves together in a quart of water for 4 hours. Chill and drink a cup or more daily.

Stinging nettle (*Urtica dioica*) is also said to be a uterine tonic that relieves stress on the kidneys and adrenals. It has high mineral and chlorophyll contents and contains calcium, phosphorus, and vitamins A and D.

Dr. Ney often prepares mixed tinctures of herbs for her patients. Some of the other herbs she includes are *Mitchella repens,* or partridge berry, another uterine tonic that relieves congestion in the pelvic organs, soothes the general nervous system, and helps to prevent miscarriage, and *Maca,* an adaptogenic herb that promotes hormonal balance, regulates the menstrual cycle, and supports energy balance. Dong quai, *Angelica sinensis,* is an adaptogen from traditional Chinese medicine; it has estrogenic properties and is used for a wide range of reproductive problems. It can cause heavy menstrual bleeding, and should not be used during pregnancy. Ashwagandha, or *Withania somnifera,* is an Ayurvedic adaptogen that helps relax the nervous system. Dr. Ney follows her patients closely, and has them stop taking *Vitex, Maca,* and *Mitchella* once they have achieved pregnancy.

Dr. Low Dog warns that if you are going to use herbs, stick with those that are considered nutritive. If they don't have a long history of use in pregnancy, you should avoid them. Some herbs stimulate menstruation; these are referred to as emmenagogues, and could make you miscarry. Herbs like chasteberry and shatavari are foodlike and considered to be safe. Many products on the market, however, are designed for sexual enhancement and fertility; these have been shown to be some of the worst offenders in terms of adulteration with less expensive substitutes, so choose cautiously and purchase only from reputable companies.

A variety of herbs have been used to treat PCOS. Dr. Low Dog recommends *shakuyaku-kanzo-to,* which is a combination of white peony root (*Paeonia lactiflora*) and licorice root. Used in traditional Chinese medicine and in Japan for fertility, it lowers testosterone and prolactin and increases progesterone. The combination restores ovulation in many women with PCOS within about three months. Exercise care with licorice; in high doses it can elevate blood pressure and cause retention of sodium and elimination of potassium. Once a woman begins ovulating, she should stop taking it; *shakuyaku-kanzo-to* is not to be taken during pregnancy.

Cinnamon can be helpful with PCOS as well. More of a lifestyle intervention than a medicine, cinnamon can increase insulin sensitivity; add ¼ teaspoon to oatmeal or yogurt. A tiny pilot study showed that 3 to 6 grams per day was effective in improving insulin sensitivity. There are two major types of cinnamon, Ceylon and Cassia; both are believed to have similar activity. To her patients with PCOS, Dr. Ney also recommends vitamin D, chromium, zinc, omega-3 fatty acids, inositol, and saw palmetto.

When considering herbs, remember that they can also be used for a wide range of other health issues that may coexist with fertility challenges; for example, herbal therapies can help you to sleep better and can aid with stress.

Detoxification

Detoxification regimens have become a fad these days. Their promoters claim that special diets, supplements, "cleanses," or even colonic irrigation can flush harmful chemicals from our bodies, leaving us rejuvenated. Many celebrities swear by their efficacy, and the endorsements just keep on coming. Is there any value to these treatments?

The first rule of detoxification is to stop ingesting toxins. This includes paying attention to the food you eat, the water you drink, the air you breathe, the chemicals you put on your skin, and any chemicals you may be exposed to at work. The good news is that growing awareness of environmental issues has created new strategies for avoidance. We can have our water tested, get a filtration system for our homes, and drink from stainless-steel water bottles. The Environmental Working Group and other agencies can help us with our food choices. Cosmetic databases evaluate tens of thousands of products, helping us make healthier selections. And federal standards require informing workers of chemicals they may be exposed to at work. These steps will markedly reduce your body burden of chemicals, and are much more important than a detox diet or product.

In addition, we can enhance our body's excretion of chemicals through judicious use of saunas, increasing our fluids and fiber intake, and eating cruciferous vegetables that rev up the liver's detoxifying ability. If you need to lose some weight before conceiving, it's best to do so slowly, because rapid weight loss results in a higher load of chemicals being mobilized from your body fat, where they are stored, into your blood. Do get the weight off and eat organic before you become pregnant; otherwise you transfer the chemicals in your body to your baby via breast milk, which contains a lot of fat. Also consider herbs such as milk thistle that help your liver to detoxify chemicals.

Dr. Ney often suggests a detoxification plan followed by a clean diet for the four months prior to attempting to conceive. She recommends that during this period women eat a whole-food, nutrient-dense diet with a lot of dark, leafy greens at every meal. She also recommends eating liver-supportive foods such as beets, carrots, and artichokes, and drinking dandelion tea—an excellent detoxifing herb. She asks all women to take probiotics, and often prescribes herbs such as milk thistle, artichoke leaf (promotes bile flow), dandelion root (a diuretic), stinging nettle, turmeric, yellow dock (anti-inflammatory herbs) and burdock (a blood purifier). Schisandra (*Schisandra chinensis*) is her all-time favorite herb. It is said to tonify and strengthen the hypothalamic, pituitary, ovarian, and adrenal organs and systems.

Dr. Low Dog recommends milk thistle for women who need to detoxify. It's very safe, even during pregnancy, and there is compelling evidence that it protects the liver cells and can help the kidneys detox as well. Schisandra, or "five-flavor fruit," can be eaten and is also safe in pregnancy. Less well-studied herbs for detoxification are *Bupleurum* and *Picrorhiza*. These should not be taken during pregnancy, but could be used in a preparatory detox plan.

Recommendations for Men

Male sperm counts have been declining for decades. While the exact cause is unknown, it is likely to be multifactorial, including environmental exposures to pesticides, endogenous estrogens, and heavy metals. Since antioxidants mitigate the effects of toxins, men who are thinking about becoming fathers should take multivitamins.

Sperm are exquisitely sensitive to oxidative stress. In the final stages of sperm formation, cytoplasm is extracted, creating a lean, fast swimmer. The cost is that with the removal of cytoplasm, some of the sperm's protection from free radicals is lost as well.

A 2010 meta-analysis reviewed thirty-four studies of more than 2,800 couples undergoing fertility treatment. When men took antioxidants, they were four times more likely than the control group to impregnate their partners, and the rate of live birth was five times higher. A wide range of antioxidants was used in the studies and included vitamins C and E, zinc, folic acid, and selenium.

Men who were treated with a combination of folic acid and zinc sulphate showed a 74 percent increase in normal sperm count. Other studies indicate that

L-arginine increases sperm count and motility; some show that zinc alone improves the sperm's motility, and there have been studies of the antioxidants vitamins C, E, and CoQ10.

The limitation of these studies is that they usually look only at sperm count and motility. Rarely do they assess pregnancy and live birth rates. When studies are funded, it is easier and less expensive, albeit less meaningful, to look at shorter-term measures such as the impact on sperm count than it is to track pregnancy and birth rates.

An antioxidant-supplement study that did look at pregnancy rates prescribed Clomid and vitamin E to men, versus Clomid alone. There was a 37 percent pregnancy rate in the partners of the men who received medication plus supplement, compared with a 13 percent pregnancy rate in the control. There was also an increase in sperm count and motility in the men who took the combination—again demonstrating the broad benefits of antioxidants.

Considering that sperm contains rich amounts of essential fatty acids, omega-3 has been looked at in men. One study compared the sperm of eighty-two infertile men with reduced sperm count to the sperm of seventy-eight fertile men. Fertile men had higher blood and spermatozoa levels of omega-3 fatty acids, compared with the infertile men. This provides presumptive evidence of the importance of omega-3. Some animal studies show that when omega-3s are given to males, they are concentrated in the sperm. Omega-3s contribute to the sperm's fluidity necessary for it to penetrate and fertilize the egg.

Vitamin D is also important for men. There is preliminary evidence that a vitamin D deficiency corresponds to an increased risk of autism in the child. Vitamin D is important in repairing DNA damage and protecting against oxidative stress, so men, too, should be sure their levels are normal.

Dr. Low Dog recommends *Tribulus terrestris,* or puncturevine, as a male reproductive tonic. Open clinical trials found that protodioscin, a compound in the leaf and fruit of *Tribulus,* can enhance sexual arousal and improve erectile dysfunction. She also notes that maca (*Maca lepidium*) is valued in South America for its fertility effects, especially in men. In the Andes, maca is eaten like a starchy tuber, and is quite safe. Dr. Low Dog recommends taking 3 grams of extract per day, or 6 to 12 grams of ground powdered maca. In addition, she recommends ginseng for erectile dysfunction. Studies done on red or white Asian ginseng (*Panax ginseng*) reveal that it increases nitric oxide, leading to improved blood flow to the penis. In Asian folklore, ginseng is used to help men maintain their fertility into old age. It is also a potent adaptogen that helps men with stress.

It is clear that dietary supplements for men and women—especially multivitamins, folic acid, vitamin D, and omega-3, and, in addition for women, iron—are beneficial during preparation for pregnancy. Please do your research before you get to the store. There are rows and rows of shelves filled with products, and it can be confusing to know which to select. In addition to the resources in this book, a trusted healthcare professional is likely to give better information than the clerk in the store. If you are on prescribed or over-the-counter medicine, ask your doctor or pharmacist about possible interactions. Read labels with care, and remember, "buyer beware" is an appropriate attitude in this relatively underregulated arena.

CHAPTER FIVE

ENVIRONMENT

I n addition to being mindful about what we put into our bodies, we need to be aware of the potential toxins in the environment in which our bodies reside. Often, protecting ourselves can seem overwhelming and beyond our control. Government agencies, including the EPA, are underfunded, and too many companies are left to self-regulate. Sometimes people simply throw up their hands and say, "The problem is everywhere; there's nothing I can do," and give up. However, the hopeful news is that, at this moment in time, a tremendous amount of information and resources exist that allow us to make wise environmental choices. These options protect our health, our hormones, and our unborn children.

In this chapter, I recommend that you follow the precautionary principle "If there is good scientific information that an action or policy *may* harm the public or the environment, then even in the absence of conclusive proof that the action or policy is harmful, the burden falls upon those taking the action or making the policy to demonstrate that it *will not* be harmful." In other words, this tells us to err on the side of caution and acknowledges the interconnectivity between the health of people and our planet. We already do this in other parts of our lives—when we

103

buckle our seat belts or lay an infant faceup in the crib. I will recommend that, when in doubt, you avoid substances and situations that might be detrimental to you or your baby.

There are several reasons to attend to environmental chemicals when you are planning a pregnancy. The first is that many environmental toxins are endocrine disruptors. This means that they can interfere with the production, release, transport, metabolism, binding, action, or elimination of hormones in the body. Specifically, they can alter levels and actions of estrogen, androgen, and thyroid—the most essential hormones for becoming pregnant as well as for steering the development of the fetus in the womb.

Another reason is that exposing a fetus to these chemicals in your womb can have much longer-term effects on your child's health. Your child may suffer from learning disabilities, hypospadias, undescended testicles, and childhood cancers; later, in adulthood, these early-life exposures can increase the risk for diabetes; heart disease; and breast, vaginal, testicular, and other cancers. Pioneers in the new field of health care research called fetal origins contend that the nine months of pregnancy may permanently influence the wiring of the brain and shape our children's susceptibility to a wide range of diseases.

Several studies have shown that babies are born having already been exposed to chemicals while in their mother's wombs. One of the most recent was conducted by the Environmental Working Group and Rachel's Network. They tested ten babies in five different states between December 2007 and June 2008 and found *an average* of 232 different chemicals in the babies' umbilical blood. This means that before your baby has taken a single breath of air, he or she has likely been exposed to extensive environmental toxins—so it is worth considering what you can do to reduce this exposure.

Around eighty thousand chemicals are registered for use with the EPA, and the impact of most of them has never been studied; in particular, they have not been researched in combination. We are subjected to these chemicals daily in the food we eat, the cosmetics we put on our bodies, the household products we use, via our furniture and carpeting, and even in the air we breathe. These multiple exposures lead to a substantial burden of chemicals in our bodies. Some (phthalates and BPA) we can easily excrete, so when we avoid them, our body burden goes down; others are more persistent, making avoidance even more critical. Ideally, legislative changes would be employed to reduce exposures, but this has been a long time coming.

A number of studies have examined how widely chemicals are distributed in our bodies. A 2006 Maine body burden study tested thirteen adults for seventy-one compounds. Given Maine's reputation as a pristine state, its citizens who participated found the results shocking. Altogether, forty-six different chemicals were identified in samples of blood, urine, and hair. On average, each participant had thirty-six toxic chemicals in his or her body. Exposures came from everyday products such as plastic containers, toys, furniture, fabric, automobiles, TVs and stereos, water bottles, medical supplies, and personal products such as shampoo, lotions, and perfume. Some of the chemicals included phthalates from cosmetics and vinyl plastic, brominated flame retardants (PBDEs) from televisions and furniture, Teflon chemicals from non-stick coatings, Bisphenol A from reusable water bottles, and metals such as lead, mercury, and arsenic.

We are just beginning to develop research methods that study the impact of synergism. The daunting message is that multiple exposures to low levels of environmental chemicals impair your health and place your baby at risk. The positive perspective focuses on the multiple benefits that a healthy lifestyle exerts. For example, when you manage stress more effectively, you not only improve the function of your hypothalamic-pituitary-ovarian axis, but also strengthen your immune response and bolster the detoxification systems of your body.

I share this research not to scare you, but to raise your awareness so that you can change your habits if necessary. Toxic chemicals are found in products we use every day. As individuals, we can make choices that create safer home and work environments and that reduce exposure to these chemicals.

Try Not to Feel Overwhelmed

Because the idea of trying to eliminate toxins from our environments can seem overwhelming, I advise you to focus on the things that you do daily or often. For example, you probably spend eight hours or more asleep in your bedroom, so that space deserves your attention. You may also spend eight hours a day in your office, so what you're exposed to there is worth considering. I advise paying more attention to the things that you do frequently, and over which you have control. If you focus here, you won't feel constantly fearful about every single thing lurking in the environment.

My colleague Dr. Joanne Perron, who is an ob-gyn at the Program on Reproductive Health and the Environment, University of California, San Francisco and a graduate of our fellowship, finds that people tend to have one of two tendencies when it comes to environmental concerns: they behave like Chicken Little, worrying that the sky is falling and predicting the worst possible outcomes, or they become paralyzed and stick their heads in the sand. "We need to find some kind of balance; otherwise the stress of worrying about it will prevent you from getting pregnant, or if you do conceive, the stress will be transmitted to your fetus," she says. "We simply cannot worry about the zillions of chemicals that exist. Instead, we should figure out our most common routes of exposure and try to eliminate them."

Another colleague, Dr. David Wallinga, who is one of the nation's leaders in environmental policy issues, and senior advisor in Science, Food, and Health at the Institute for Agriculture and Trade Policy, suggests that people change the way they think about pregnancy, urging them to consider pregnancy an opportunity to create the first environment their children will inhabit. As he says, "That approach will bear fruit, not only when the baby is born, but throughout the life of the child. There is no magic bullet; it's a process, and you can't get overwhelmed. It's best to start with baby steps that add up quickly in terms of creating the healthiest environment that you can. Small steps do make a difference."

Environmental Chemicals and Your Child

Before I move into specific recommendations, I want to explain why a fetus, infant, and small child are at such great risk—in fact, at much greater risk than adults. It is due in part to the concept of critical windows of susceptibility. A fetus (or young child) is still developing its neurological system, which makes it exquisitely sensitive to chemicals. Its immune system is not fully developed; therefore, its ability to protect itself is limited. And its detoxification systems have not fully matured, so it is less able to metabolize and excrete chemicals. While the placenta offers some protection against unwanted chemical exposures during fetal life, it is not an effective barrier against environmental pollutants. Many metals, for instance, easily cross the placenta, and the mercury concentration in umbilical cord blood can be substantially higher than in maternal blood. The blood-brain barrier, which protects the adult brain from many toxic chemicals, is not completely formed until about six months after birth. Thus a fetus or young child needs to be guarded more carefully against toxins than a grown-up does.

What to Do About What We Eat

As I mentioned in Chapter 3, "Nutrition," for the average person, the greatest exposure to chemicals is through food. This is one of the more manageable concerns, as we can use a myriad of resources to make smart choices. As discussed, the Dirty Dozen and Clean 15 lists can help you to minimize intake of toxins in fruits and vegetables. The Environmental Working Group (www.ewg.org) calculates that if you buy fruits and vegetables from the Clean 15 rather than the Dirty Dozen, you can reduce your exposure to pesticides by 92 percent. Strawberries, usually one of the worst offenders, have more than fifty pesticide residues, so that is a fruit you definitely want to buy organic or skip altogether. I'd recommend that you eat the fruits and vegetables on the Dirty Dozen list only if you can find organic; on the other hand, the Clean 15 have so little residue that conventional is just fine.

The EPA has identified seventy-three suspect pesticides with hormone-disrupting effects; Beyond Pesticides has a list of these chemicals (www.beyondpesticides.org). Several studies have shown that if you feed young children an entirely organic diet, the amount of pesticides in their urine goes down dramatically, and almost immediately. In other words, avoidance works, does so quickly, and lowers your body burden of pesticides.

Next, let's talk about fish. As discussed in "Nutrition," fish is an important part of our diets as it contains fatty acids that promote optimal brain development in babies. On the other hand, eating too much fish can put your baby at risk of neurological problems. This dilemma often troubles patients of mine who want to do what's best for their children. One patient, Jonathan, explained to me that he and his wife were raised in kosher homes. Early in their marriage, they moved to the Midwest. Lacking a kosher butcher, they began eating a lot of fish for protein. He wonders, now, whether his older daughter's autism might have been a result. This, he relates sadly, preceded the FDA warnings about eating fish during pregnancy.

While you should not skip fish altogether, please do avoid fish high in mercury and PCBs. Smaller fish and fish that feed on plants or algae will have less contamination than those that are big or carnivorous (because they bioaccumulate more toxins). Use sites such as that of the Monterey Bay Aquarium to help choose fish that are high in omega-3s and low in mercury and PCBs. Some companies specialize in selling smaller fish—another way to reduce exposure. Dr. Perron adds that ob-gyns often neglect to tell women to take the skin off fish before cooking. Since this is where most of the organopollutants reside, deskinning is a healthful move.

Persistent organopollutants (POPs) are chemicals that were frequently used by manufacturers from the 1940s to the 1970s, when they were for the most part banned by Congress. These include PCBs, DDT, and anything containing a halogen molecule (like chlorine or bromine). Synthetic halogens were added to the chemicals to help prevent breakdown; an unintended side effect, however, was that these chemicals "persist" in the environment in soil and water, and are eventually absorbed and stored in animal fats. When we eat fatty meats, we take in pesticides from the grains as well as legacy chemicals (which essentially never go away) that are in the soil and the water that the animals consume. The more you can omit animal fats, the more you will eliminate these halogens, which are endocrine disruptors that affect thyroid function as well as fetal brain development. Additional strategies to reduce POPs include choosing leaner cuts of meat and removing the skin from poultry. When you do eat lean meat, eating organic will further reduce hormone, antibiotic, and pesticide exposure.

Presumptive evidence links POPs in the mother's body with changes in the fetal brain, resulting in ADHD, autism, or reduced IQ. This is another reason (besides the Nurses' Health Study II, which showed that swapping about an ounce of animal protein for the same amount of plant protein reduced the risk of ovulatory infertility by 50 percent) that you'll want to get more protein from plant foods when you are pregnant.

Keep in mind that grazing cows and free-range chickens are exposed to legacy chemicals in soil and water, so it's still best not to eat a lot of animal fat, even if it is organic.

Packaging

Perhaps you've never given much thought to how your food is packaged. Now is the time, as this is another potential source of exposure to environmental chemicals that you can control. BPA is in many of our plastic water bottles. It doesn't take too long to develop the habit of carrying your own stainless-steel water bottle. You can fill it at home with filtered water, save a lot of money, and reduce the burden to the environment of all those plastic bottles.

Plastic wrap can leach into foods, so unwrap cheeses and other items as soon as you get them home from the grocery store. (You can use parchment paper to rewrap and then place in containers.) The safest plastic wraps contain low-density polyethylene (LDPE); these include Glad Cling Wrap or Handi-Wrap and Saran Premium Wrap. And don't ever microwave in plastic—use glass or ceramic instead. The reason to avoid phthalates (plasticizers used as solvents and also to make plastics more flexible) is that they are endocrine disruptors that affect parents and babies alike. Studies have shown that men exposed to higher levels of phthalates have lower sperm counts, altered sperm quality, and significantly lower levels of testosterone.

Cans are another package to be wary of. The lining of almost all our canned foods contains bisphenol A (BPA), an endocrine disruptor that has been linked to increased miscarriages as well as obesity, early onset of puberty, and breast and prostate cancer later in life. It also raises the risk of diabetes and heart disease. Its structure is very similar to diethylstilbestrol (DES), the synthetic estrogen given to women in order to prevent miscarriage in the first part of the twentieth century, until it was discovered to cause birth defects. BPA may be even stronger than natural estrogen. Over 90 percent of Americans show signs of it in their bodies when tested. Sadly, infants often have some of the highest levels because it's in their baby bottles (unless you buy BPA-free or use glass) and in the liners of infant formula cans.

You can make a difference by knowing which cans are the worst offenders. The Breast Cancer Research Foundation tested three hundred of them and found cans used for coconut milk, soups, meat, vegetables, fish, beans, meal replacements, and fruits to have the highest levels of BPA. Some natural food companies have gone the extra mile to use BPA-free cans. They cost about 14 percent over market rate, and speak to the companies' commitment to health. The following site lists BPA-free packaging: www.treehugger.com/files/2010/03/7-bpa-free-canned-foods.php.

Before you get too discouraged, let me share the findings of a 2011 study published in Environmental Health Perspectives. Five (lucky) families had all their meals prepared for them from fresh, organic ingredients and avoided BPA-containing food packaging. Over just a three-day period, average BPA levels, measured in urine samples, dropped by 60 percent, and the participants with the highest exposure levels saw a 75 percent reduction. Phthalate urine levels dropped by more than 50 percent as well. A 2010 study had similarly hopeful results. In this second trial, aptly named the Temple Stay study, twenty-five people lived in a Buddhist monastery for five days, ate the same vegetarian diet as the monks, and followed their daily practices. All showed reduced levels of phthalates, pesticides, and antibiotic residues in their urine.

Advice in the nutrition chapter bears repeating here: eat less processed and refined food, which is typically higher in fats and added sugars and has more additives and chemicals. By preparing your own food, as was done in the first study, you also avoid packaging that can leach hormonally active chemicals.

A few last words about your food: utensils. For cooking, it is better to use cast iron, stainless steel, or ceramic, as nonstick pans can be a source of Teflon chemicals. Get yourself a French press if you drink coffee to avoid the plastic tubing that the water usually runs through. Lastly, use glass or ceramics in the microwave instead of plastic, as warmer temperatures increase the rate at which chemicals leach into food and drinks. Also use these same materials to store your food, especially if the foods are fatty or acidic, which, like heat, increases the absorption of the chemicals.

How to Make Sure that Your Water Is Safe

Question: which is better for your health—bottled water or tap? The answer may surprise many of you. It's probably tap, for two reasons. Tap water is regulated by the Environmental Protection Agency (EPA), whereas bottled water is not. Your municipal systems must pay a certified lab to test samples weekly, monthly, and quarterly, for a long list of contaminants. Bottled water that crosses state lines is considered a food product, and is overseen by the Food and Drug Administration (FDA), but their standards are less stringent. For instance, they require water bottlers to perform tests as infrequently as once a year.

Often people think that when they drink bottled water, they're getting pure stuff, but actually much of it is simply municipal water (i.e., tap water) that has been packaged. In addition, phthalates and BPA in the plastic water bottles can leach into your water. In general, avoid drinking packaged water unless you carefully check out the water's origins (for instance, a pristine spring), and drink it only from glass or other nonplastic containers.

Well water, too, can contain harmful contaminates. Since arsenic, heavy metals, and radon can be naturally present in the groundwater, it is important to have your well water tested annually by a specialist. Depending on what is found, an appropriate filtration system can be added.

So what's wrong with drinking tap water? After all, the EPA regulates more than a hundred pollutants through the 1972 Clean Water Act, and strictly limits ninety-one chemicals or contaminants in tap water through the Safe Drinking Water Act. The problems include enforcement and the by-products of disinfection. The combination of chlorine, or other halogens, plus organic material in water supplies creates "disinfection by-products" that exceed safe limits. In addition, vaporized chlorine and disinfection by-products are inhaled in the shower. Furthermore, water treatment facilities have difficulty in making sure that fluoride levels are carefully regulated. In the West and Southwest, perchlorate (think rocket fuel) is another contaminant.

Nathan Daley, MD, a graduate of our fellowship who practices integrative and ecological preventive medicine in Colorado, points out that not only is municipal water chlorine treated, it can also contain cadmium, lead, or even bacteria. A 2009 exposé in *The New York Times* stated that the EPA is failing because they cannot police our water. In it, EPA administrator Lisa Jackson acknowledged that "the nation's water does not meet public health goals, and enforcement of water pollution laws is unacceptably low." The *Times* assembled data from across the nation; by going to www.nytimes.com/toxicwaters, you can see how water in your municipality fares. Sadly, it is estimated that one in ten Americans has been exposed to drinking water that contains dangerous chemicals or fails to meet federal health benchmarks.

The good news is that a solution is available, at least on an individual level. Because of the many failures in our municipal water system, add your own layer of protection by filtering water before you drink it. Use this filtered tap water for drinking and cooking, and carry it with you in a stainless-steel or glass water bottle. It's best to use a reverse-osmosis filter for drinking water; it removes elemental products such as uranium and cadmium as well as fluoride. The downside is that the process wastes a lot of water, so it is not recommended for bathing. You can take the additional step of filtering all of your household water with a charcoal filter to avoid inhaling toxic vapors while showering.

Personal Care Products

It makes sense to investigate products that you use every day to find out whether or not you have made good choices. While it takes a bit of work, you need to research and select products only every couple of years. Here's what I do: when I need to buy an item, I go on www.ewg.org/skindeep, the extensive database kept by the Environmental Working Group. I look up my current product, and if it rates well, in the range of 2 or lower, I buy it again. If not, I look for an alternative. The rating system is 0–2, low hazard; 3–6, moderate; 7–10, high. When you click on the product, it will tell you what the environmental hazards are.

Even within one brand, products can range from very safe to not at all safe, so it's really worth checking out the shampoo, cosmetics, moisturizer, sunscreen, and any other products that you use frequently. If you don't have a favorite brand, you can search for a safer one on the skindeep site. Make a list of the products with the fewest chemicals to bring with you to the store.

Here's another challenge: *organic* on a cosmetic product label doesn't mean much. The FDA does not have the authority to regulate cosmetics; only organic food is carefully regulated. Similarly, terms like *natural* and *hypoallergenic* are marketing terms with no "teeth." Your best strategy is to look up the ingredients yourself. The Campaign for Safe Cosmetics site (www.safecosmetics.org) and the Environmental Working Group site (www.ewg.org/skindeep) are two useful sites.

Fragrances are chemicals used in perfumes, body lotions, and shampoos, as well as in scented candles and in car or room deodorizers. Companies do not have to disclose what the fragrances contain, as the ingredients are considered "trade secrets." Unless the label says pure essential oils, it is probably worth avoiding all scented (and even many unscented) products. They contain phthalates, neurotoxins, and synthetic musks, most of which are endocrine disruptors. Synthetic musks such as Galaxolyde and Tonalyde are persistent; they don't break down well in the environment, and they can bioaccumulate in our fat. In a study that looked at breast milk, *every* woman tested had at least one type of synthetic musk, while 82 percent of the women had at least two kinds of musk in their breast milk. So obviously it's best to avoid these items that contain fragrance and that can interfere with the proper working of the hormonal system.

Cleaning Products

Household cleaning products also contribute to your body burden of industrial chemicals. Cleaning solvents are oxidative stressors and can affect the mitochondria, developing immune cells, and DNA in the fetus. Dr. Wallinga points out that choosing environmentally conscious products reduces the number of choices available, making it easier to select. You can avoid using toxic cleaning chemicals and save money by switching to a combination of baking soda and vinegar, or other green alternatives. (Alice's Wonder Spray is one such option—see Additional Resources.)

Use a HEPA filter in your vacuum so that pollutants are removed from the dust. Dr. Daley points out that vacuuming the carpet stirs dust laden with chemicals up into the air. He adds, "It's great if the man can do a lot of the cleaning when his partner is pregnant."

The Air You Breathe

Steer clear of vehicle and smokestack emissions, the most common kinds of air pollution. Polycyclic aromatic hydrocarbons (PAH) are chemicals that occur in crude oil, coal, and gas. Pregnant women exposed to PAHs have shorter gestations and their babies have lower birth weights, smaller head circumferences, developmental delays, and, later in life, an increased risk of cancer. In addition to car and bus exhaust, these pollutants are found in emissions from residential heating and power sources. Advising to avoid breathing car and bus exhaust states the obvious. Less obvious tips include not sitting in the back of a bus, not idling your car when you stop for something, and not breathing the fumes while pumping at the gas station. Also, when driving in traffic, once you air out the car, roll up your window and use the air-recirculation button, which blocks 99 percent of exhaust from the cars in front of you.

To improve indoor air quality, use high MERV (minimum efficiency reporting value)–rated air filters (a rating of 12 to 15) for your heating, ventilation, and air conditioning systems. These filters are very effective in removing dust, pollen, and chemical pollutants. In smaller rooms of up to 400 square feet (think your bedroom or office), you can use stand-alone HEPA filters, which remove up to 99 percent of particles from the air. Avoid using air fresheners in your car or home. Even "unscented" or "all-natural" fresheners can contain phthalates, used to make the scent linger longer on your skin or in the air, as well as synthetic musks.

Insecticides and Pesticides

While it may be second nature for you to grab a can of spray when you see a bug in your home or office, this is another practice that you can modify. The Columbia Center for Children's Environmental Health conducted an important study with twenty-five healthy pregnant women living in the Bronx or Manhattan. Rather than using chemical insecticides, the women employed integrated pest management strategies, such as sticky traps, bait stations, and gels; plugging cracks with caulk; and filling big holes with steel wool. With these methods, they reduced the cockroaches by half, and essentially eliminated toxic pesticides as measured in blood samples of the mothers and their babies at birth. This small study shows one effective way to reduce chemicals in your body.

Maternal exposure to domestic pesticides (as in weed killers, ant and roach sprays, flea dips and collars, and mosquito sprays) is associated with childhood leukemia. These chemical exposures may also contribute to low birth weight, neurodevelopmental and birth defects, pregnancy loss, and infertility. Men exposed to pesticides and solvents have lower sperm counts. A study of men living in agricultural areas in Missouri revealed that they had 40 percent lower counts and higher urine levels of pesticides than men in urban areas.

Also avoid spraying weed killers, fungicides, and pesticides outside your home, and take off your shoes before you enter the house, so you don't bring in dust laden with pesticides. At the very least, use a doormat to remove dust from your shoes when you enter. Dr. Wallinga points out that lawn chemicals are not well tested for safety. As he says, "None of us should expect the perfect lawn. Yes, your lawn may have a few weeds, but there will be no chemicals that would impact your or your baby's health." You may want to follow the strategy used in the New York City study; use integrative pest management to reduce domestic exposure and forgo the chemicals on your lawn.

Avoiding EMF Exposures

In modern society, we use a wide range of products that emit electromagnetic fields (EMFs). We can't avoid EMFs entirely, but we can minimize unnecessary exposure. If you have a wireless modem, consider unplugging it at night. Don't place the wireless next to the baby's room, or indeed in any bedrooms. And no one should actually use a laptop on their lap—put it on a table instead. Survey your work and home environments for machines that may emit large fields.

In May 2011, the World Health Organization classified cell phones in the same way they do lead, chloroform, and engine exhaust—as potential carcinogens. They were particularly worried about increases in two types of brain tumors. In 2008, a study at the Cleveland Clinic of 361 men treated at a fertility clinic revealed that men who used their cell phones more than four hours each day had the lowest average sperm count and motility, and the lowest numbers of normal, viable sperm. While we may all be better off keeping cell phones at a distance from our ears, men may also wish to increase the distance from their genitals. There is evidence that men have more abnormal sperm morphology when they wear their phones on their bodies or keep them in their pockets near their reproductive organs.

The risk of exposure to your cell phone's electromagnetic field drops exponentially if you're just a short distance away from it, so use your speaker, and don't wear it on your body. Also avoid Bluetooth, which has an EMF of its own, and rather than holding your cell phone next to your ear, use a cord. There is a concern that wired headsets can act as antennas for the phone and actually increase EMFs very focally at the ear. The type of headset that has been shown to reduce EMFs at the head to near zero are the hollow tube ("air tube") headsets. For more information, go to www.ewg .org/cellphoneradiation/Bluetooth-Cell-Cordless-Phones.

Finally, you can investigate the specific absorption rate (SAR), or the amount of radiofrequency energy absorbed from the phone into the local tissues. Kudos to the city of San Francisco, which now requires that SAR be disclosed when the phone is sold.

Additional Environmental Actions to Consider

Furniture and carpets follow a parabolic curve when they are off-gassing. This means that when you first bring the new item into your home, there is a very high release of chemicals. This decreases quickly over the first few weeks, then low levels of off-gassing continue for months or years. (Some of these products may release more gases as they degrade.) When planning a pregnancy, either avoid buying new furniture and carpet or buy green products instead. In addition, consider buying formaldehyde-free cribs and an organic mattress for your baby. For more information, go to www .healthybuildingnetwork.org.

Lead in paint was banned in 1978, and in gasoline in 1996. Most exposure to lead today comes from old paint, as well as contaminated water and soil. Lead is one of the most toxic substances to fetal development; it can cause neurological impairment, mental retardation, and kidney damage. If your house is old and has lead paint, it's best to cover it with fresh paint without removing the old coat, since removing paint releases lead into the air; it then settles in dust, which you then inhale. In addition, avoid remodeling projects when preparing to conceive or when pregnant, and if you must paint, use no-VOC paint, which is better than low-VOC.

Check for items embedded with flame retardants, or polybrominated diphenyl ethers (PBDEs), and eliminate them from your home. PBDEs are organopollutants and may be endocrine disruptors and developmental neurotoxicants. A 2010 study found that each tenfold increase in the blood concentration of four PBDE chemicals was linked to a 30 percent decrease in the odds of becoming pregnant each month. In addition to being in furniture, PBDEs could be in your nursing pillow, infant car seat, televisions, electronics, computers, upholstery, carpeting, or synthetic clothing. Because PBDEs are so prevalent in household dust, wet mopping when dusting and frequent hand washing, particularly before eating, can help to reduce exposure.

Should I Be Tested for Toxins?

Many women ask me if they should be tested for toxins before they conceive. One challenge is that the tests used in body burden studies cost thousands of dollars to carry out. A second is that some toxins are stored in parts of the body where blood and urine tests may not detect them. Finally, there is the question of what you will do with the results of the tests. If you feel you can make the changes suggested in this chapter on your own, I encourage you to do so. If you feel you'll be inspired to make changes in your lifestyle only by knowing the results of the tests, then they may be worth the investment.

One test to consider is for mercury. Increased blood levels suggest a relatively recent exposure to the toxin, while a twenty-four-hour urine sample gives more of an average past history of exposure to metallic or inorganic mercury. Especially if you are a sushi-lover or have been eating fish known to be high in mercury, a twenty-four-hour urine test is the best way to go. Being tested would indicate whether you need to go off fish altogether or if what you're currently eating is safe.

At present, very few labs test for environmental chemicals and those that do, primarily do the testing only for scientific studies. (This is partly because they must create a sterile environment clear of their own pollutants and it is too time-consuming and costly for one person at a time.) Commonweal biomonitoring resource center director Sharyle Patton hopes that in the future, individual biomonitoring will be available. She believes the data could be used to point scientific studies in the most critical direction and help corporations reformulate products as well as monitor laws limiting exposures.

CHAPTER 6

MIND-BODY MEDICINE

We talk about the mind and the body, or the body and the mind, as if they were completely separate entities, but this is a false dichotomy. We know that everything you experience in your mind affects your body, and vice versa. Our language is full of phrases that identify the intimate connection between our emotions and our physical bodies: we talk about heartache or when something is breaking our back because, intuitively, we know this connection exists.

We regularly access the mind-body connection, although we don't necessarily speak of it in these terms. Mind-body describes the power of the mind to influence the body, and the body to influence the mind. Worry is an example of the mind influencing the body. In this case, our imagination about what might occur frightens us. Physically, this can be accompanied by a rapid heart rate; a sinking sensation in the pit of our stomach; and rapid, shallow breathing. Anyone who has been frightened by a horror movie has experienced how the mind can change the body's physiology.

Imagery can also be used for healing, as described later in this chapter. Alternatively, we can mobilize the body to settle the mind. A deep sigh is an unconscious way to reset your nervous system; a full abdominal breath can be intentionally used for the same purpose. Yoga, tai chi, progressive muscle relaxation, and other physical activities can lead to a quieting of the mind and of the sympathetic nervous system. Mind-body medicine provides an incredible way to access our innate healing response, and is an important element of integrative medicine.

That the mind-body connection is so powerful is revealed in the need for placebos in clinical studies. Placebos show the power of belief to create changes in our physiology. Just being in a study, having attention paid to us, and having a researcher suggest that we can get better, has been shown to lead to up to 80 percent improvement in some conditions. (Blood sugar is minimally susceptible to placebo, whereas depression falls at the high end of placebo response.) Placebos demonstrate that we can use the mind to turn on a healing response, to reduce pain, and even to settle an overactive immune system.

As an example, one of my patients had unexplained pain in his leg. His physical exam, lab work, and X-rays were all normal. When I asked him to tell me a bit more about his life, he explained that he'd just had to kick his alcoholic son out of his house. As soon as he spoke the words, it became apparent to him that the emotional fallout had resulted in his having a literal pain in his leg. As the stress of the situation with his son dissipated, so, too, did his physical discomfort.

Many women find mind-body medicine techniques helpful during their fertility quests. Suzanne, a former social worker who is now a stay-at-home mom, describes here how she learned to use mind-body skills to help her conceive:

> In October 2008, when I was twenty-seven, my husband, Billy (who is an oncologist), and I decided that we were ready to start a family after being married for two years. I had ovarian cysts when I was young, which were treated with the pill. Then once they were resolved, I stayed on it.
>
> Even before I went off the pill, I was afraid that I would have trouble conceiving. I had a few friends who'd had fertility issues, and I just had a feeling about it. But Billy felt that we'd be fine. The first time I got my period after going off the pill, I had a twenty-eight-day cycle, but then the next cycle was forty days. I saw an ob-gyn in

November and sat in his office and cried; I thought something was wrong with me, and I was afraid I wouldn't be able to get pregnant. The doctor explained exactly how you get pregnant; I'd had a course in human sexuality in college, but even then I didn't quite realize that there were only a couple of days a month when you could conceive. I felt better after seeing him, but then I had another forty-day cycle. A voice in the back of my mind said that something was wrong.

In April 2009, I went to a fertility clinic and was told that I had PCOS and wouldn't be able to get pregnant on my own. They gave me letrozole (an ovulation-inducing medication) in order to make me ovulate. The doctor was very flippant because I was young and wasn't overweight. He said I'd do one of three things: get pregnant; get frustrated and come back again right away; or wait six months and then come back. He didn't even tell me about ovulation predictor kits. First I had to take Provera to have a period, but it gave me suicidal thoughts, which was terrifying. I then took letrozole to try to make my body ovulate, but this did not work. A good friend told me to get a twenty-one-day progesterone drawn to see if the letrozole worked, and this was how we knew I failed that drug. I switched doctors within the same practice and my new physician prescribed Clomid. We tried this for two cycles, first 50 mg and then 100 mg, and I still didn't ovulate. The waiting was the hardest part; you wait for your period to come, and then you get the heartbreak of the Clomid not working. The waiting was absolutely horrible.

I needed something to help me deal with the stress, so I began seeing a counselor who taught me self-hypnosis. It helped me to relax and sleep better, and also to work on some other issues that I needed to deal with. She taught me to imagine my family's vacation home and touch my fingers together to go into a trance. I could not have done it by myself, but it was easy with her help. I did it a few times a day, and the more I practiced, the easier it became. I got to a point where I could do it while waiting to see the doctor, or waiting

121

for the ultrasound. I could put myself into a trance and then relax about the doctor visits. I saw the counselor for six months. Later, when I finally ovulated, my therapist told me to write a script visualizing the sperm and egg meeting. When I ovulated, I would recite to myself, "The sperm has free access to my egg. The healthy egg and healthy sperm join together. As one, they make their way down my fallopian tube into my uterus, where they safely implant. The embryo is safe and healthy in my uterus."

I also did acupuncture, and had a massage once a month. I joined an online support group, which was very helpful, too. In addition, I started to exercise and tried to eat more healthily.

I switched practices after three failed cycles, and the new doctor put me on 200 mg of Clomid, double what I had been taking. I finally felt that I had found a doctor who took time with me and understood my feelings. She did not minimize our struggle as the other doctors had. I took Provera for a week to start my period, then Clomid for days 3–7, then had an ultrasound on day 12. The ultrasound showed that there were two small follicles, and I ovulated on day 21. When I went in to see the doctor, I'd had a negative home pregnancy test, and I demanded that she give me a plan for the next six months. She said, "Have you considered that you might be pregnant despite the negative test? It might have been too soon." I went home and took another test, and this time it showed that I was indeed pregnant. This was in September 2009, one year after I went off the pill. I had a good pregnancy and long labor, but a fine delivery. Our son was born in June 2010 when I was twenty-nine.

Without the self-hypnosis and acupuncture, I wouldn't have survived emotionally. People would say to me, "You have to relax," and I'd want to scream. I wasn't making eggs, so it wasn't about relaxing. Or people would thoughtlessly mention, "Oh, I got pregnant while I was on the pill." You want to blame yourself; was I bad in some way? Or is it that I wouldn't be a good mother? Once I told Billy, "You can call it quits if we can't have a baby." He said, "Of course not; we will have children one way or another."

Going through this was the hardest thing I've ever done; you feel as if something has been stolen from you. However, I feel that going through this struggle made me a better mother; I don't get as upset about things, and I'm calmer and more grateful for our son than if it had been easy for me to get pregnant. This time around when we try to have a second baby, I will be more open and talk about it with people. The message that I want to convey to other women is, you're not alone, and don't be embarrassed if you have trouble getting pregnant. A lot of people are in the same boat.

The Physiology of Stress

We all experience stress in our lives. We certainly know how it feels to be stressed—whether we experience it as a sense of distress, a feeling of anxiety, or symptoms in the body such as tension headaches, irritable bowel syndrome, or an upset stomach. But we may be less aware of the impact moment to moment on our physiology, or longer term on our health. Here I will briefly outline the changes that occur in your body when you feel stressed. Then, in greater detail, I will review the physiology of stress and its impact on reproductive hormones.

Our nervous system is divided into two parts: one half, the sympathetic nervous system, activates the stress response in our bodies; the other half, the parasympathetic nervous system, is responsible for our relaxation responses. The sympathetic nervous system (SNS) is sometimes called the fight-or-flight reaction. In primitive times, it prepared us to flee from or fight predators. In times of distress, the SNS increases heart rate, raises blood pressure, and contracts blood vessels, which, long ago, enabled us to better fight to protect ourselves or to run from danger.

Physiologically, the parasympathetic nervous system is the counterpoise to the SNS; it slows the heart rate and increases digestion and intestinal activities. It is sometimes referred to as the "rest and digest" side of the nervous system. Together, 123 the sympathetic and parasympathetic are called the autonomic nervous system because they function automatically. You experience this all the time: without conscious direction, your gut digests your food, your heart beats, and your lungs breathe.

In addition to the autonomic nervous system, hormones play a role in regulating the stress responses of our bodies. Hormones are chemical messages sent by a gland (including the pituitary in the brain, the thyroid in the neck, and adrenals in the abdomen) that signal other parts of the body and direct them to action. One function of hormones is to signal the body when it is overly stressed. To do so, it activates the most prominent stress hormone, cortisol, which is produced by the adrenals.

Stress hormones are potent signals to the ovaries and testes, too. From an evolutionary perspective, this interdependence makes perfect sense: if a woman is under great stress, it would not be an optimal time for her to become pregnant. Biologically, this is the time to focus upon survival rather than reproduction. The multiple hormonal feedback loops signal both men's and women's organs during times of stress as if to say, "Wrong time to think about conceiving."

Here's how it works. Reproductive hormonal signaling normally begins in a portion of the brain called the hypothalamus. Initially, the hypothalamus secretes gonadotropic-releasing hormones (GnRH), which send a message to the pituitary gland to produce luteinizing and follicle-stimulating hormones (LH and FSH). LH and FSH in turn signal the ovaries and the testes to produce the hormones estrogen, progesterone, and testosterone.

In women, FSH stimulates the growth of follicular granulosa cells and the production of estrogen. LH controls the maturation of the egg, as well as ovulation and luteinization in the follicles. (Luteinization is the process in which an ovarian follicle, having expelled its egg, changes into the corpus luteum and begins to secrete progesterone.)

When the level of estrogen and progesterone produced by the ovaries reaches a certain point, the body sends signals back to the pituitary, which in turn reduce secretion of LH and FSH. This creates a bi-directional feedback loop that begins with the hypothalamus and pituitary sending signals to the ovaries, and continues with the ovaries sending signals in the opposite direction. This beautiful dance between the glands is typical of endocrine systems.

As it turns out, stress has both a direct and an indirect effect on the brain, and also on the sexual organs in men and women. Stress acts directly on the hypothalamus by suppressing GnRH, which reduces the pituitary's secretion of LH and FSH. Similarly, in men, stress can have a negative effect on the testes, which inhibits testosterone production and the creation of sperm.

In addition, when we are stressed, the hypothalamus signals our adrenal glands to produce more hormones, called glutocorticosteroids (sometimes abbreviated as steroids or cortisol), which affect insulin, and insulin-like growth factor one. Interestingly, women have glucocorticoid receptors on their follicles, corpus luteum, and ovarian surface epithelium cells, permitting stress hormones to signal the ovaries that the timing is not right for reproduction.

Dr. Sarah Berga, professor of reproductive endocrinology and infertility at Emory University, has studied stress-induced anovulation (SIA), defined as menstrual cycles in which stress interferes with the release of an egg from the ovary. She documented that in women with SIA, there was no rise in basal body temperature or changes in cervical mucus that would signal ovulation. A more subtle pattern is functional hypothalamic amenorrhea (FHA), where women have blunted hormonal responses to FSH or GnRH. Dr. Berga's concern is that if the hypothalamic pituitary axis is disrupted, there is not only an ovarian effect but also a negative effect upon adrenal and thyroid activity. (This is because the adrenals and thyroid are also stimulated by hypothalamus and pituitary.) Dr. Berga worries that when reproductive endocrinologists address the ovaries only by using gonadotropins to stimulate them, and do not address the fact that the stress is also affecting cortisol levels and thyroid function, they are risking women's overall health and the health of their unborn children. She strongly believes that the right approach is to broadly address the stress, thereby reversing all of the hormonal abnormalities, rather than just stimulating the ovaries to produce eggs.

Dr. Berga has shown that while you can restore fertility with gonadotropin injections (drugs that stimulate the ovaries to release eggs), these injections will not correct the underlying broader, stress-induced suppression of hormone production by the pituitary gland. In contrast, Dr. Berga's research reveals that cognitive behavioral therapy (a form of psychotherapy that helps identify negative thought patterns) can

125

restore full ovarian function as well as adrenal, thyroid, and any other neuroendocrine functions. In 2003, she enrolled sixteen women with functional hypothalamic amenorrhea (i.e., no period for six months without evidence of a physical problem) in a twenty-week study. Dr. Berga measured estrogen and progesterone levels as well as vaginal bleeding. Of the ten women randomized (randomly chosen to receive one or other of the treatments being studied) to receive cognitive behavioral therapy, eight resumed ovulating. The remaining two women had partial recovery of ovarian function. Of the six women who did not receive therapy, only two experienced renewed ovarian activity. This small study suggests that cognitive behavioral therapy might be effective in restoring normal ovulation.

One surprising finding from Dr. Berga's research is that multiple small stressors had a greater effect on ovarian function than one big stressful event. She exposed monkeys to low-level psychosocial stress by moving them to new housing, and also created a moderate energy imbalance by introducing more exercise and restricting their diets. When Dr. Berga compared the impact of each individual stressor to all the stressors in combination (moving, exercising more, and limiting their diet), she found that seven out of ten monkeys had abnormal menstrual cycles with the combination, compared to only one out of ten with any single stressor. The implications are that for stress, a little of this and a little of that may have a greater biological impact than a single big stressor. This outcome is not necessarily what we'd predict, and is extremely relevant for modern life, as most women tend to experience many stressors at once and often underplay their effects.

Developing a Personal Practice

Because what we experience mentally has such a significant impact on our physical health, I strongly advocate that you develop a mind-body practice as a general life-coping skill, and even more so to relieve the stress of trying to conceive. I will teach you to access the amazing power inherent in the mind-body connection by using a variety of practices that regulate your autonomic nervous system. I'll tell you about some of my own practices, too, and describe studies that show how stress affects fertility.

I will highlight the work of two experts in mind-body medicine who've spent their careers working with women and fertility, and who lent their expertise to this chapter. The first is Dr. Alice Domar, a psychologist and one of the leading researchers in the area of stress and fertility. Domar pioneered research showing that mind-body skills groups not only relieve the stress of infertility but also enhance fertility. She is the author of *Healing Mind, Healthy Woman* and *Conquering Infertility*.

The second is Helen Adrienne, LCSW, BCD. Helen teaches mind-body stress reduction classes at the New York University Fertility Center and is the author of *On Fertile Ground: Healing Infertility.* She has two blogs: The Baby Manifest-O on her Web site, www.mind-body-unity.com, and another on *Psychology Today's,* www .psychologytoday.com/fertile-ground.

Practices and Coping Strategies

There is an incredible range of mind-body tools that are relaxing, fun, and even creative. Often I'm asked, what is the best mind-body strategy? I always say that it depends on who you are. For instance, my type A patients often have a terrible time with meditation. It's really hard for them to sit still and quiet their minds. Yoga, tai chi, or active forms of relaxation such as progressive muscle relaxation often work better. Some patients love interactive guided imagery; others feel frustrated by it, saying they just can't visualize things. (By the way, it's fine to "hear" or simply "sense" in guided imagery—"seeing" is not required.)

I usually refer people to mind-body groups. These multiple-session skill-building classes teach a wide range of strategies, including hypnosis, yoga, imagery, breath work, mindfulness, journaling, body scanning, and cognitive restructuring. The underlying purpose of exposing participants to all of these is to allow people to find a technique that truly resonates, and to make it a regular practice that can be embedded into the fabric of one's life.

As Alice Domar says, "Mind-body work is like a buffet; the first time, you want to sample everything, then go back to what works for you. You can see the practices as a toolbox, from which you can pull out whatever tool you need. Getting a negative

127

pregnancy test can require a different tool than when your mother-in-law makes a snide comment about the fact that you aren't pregnant yet."

Practices that Elicit the Relaxation Response

I am a very strong advocate for the benefits of developing a regular practice that elicits the relaxation response. Coined by Dr. Herbert Benson, with whom Dr. Domar trained, the relaxation response is the body's physiological reaction that is the opposite of the stress response.

The relaxation response is initiated by two steps:

1) a mental focus on a sound, word, phrase, or prayer; and
2) coordinating repetition with the breath.

If a sound or word is chosen, it is said either silently or aloud every time you exhale. If a phrase or prayer is chosen, half is said on the inhalation and the other half is said on the exhalation. Maintain a passive attitude of not worrying about how well you are performing; if you lose your place, just let it go and start again. This perspective, along with repetition, helps put aside distracting thoughts. As mentioned earlier, the relaxation response evokes the quieting side of our parasympathetic nervous system, counteracting the fight-or-flight reaction of the sympathetic nervous system.

With regular practice, over time, your body attunes to the signals of the relaxation response and can rapidly go to a place of deep relaxation. This results from using the practice often, so that your body instantly knows what to do. Learn and use these skills when you are not stressed; then if you are, you can quickly move into this relaxed state (as opposed to when someone tells you to "just relax," and you can't simply flip). If you have trained your body in relaxation, its ability to relax in times of stress is greatly improved because you have a well-established pathway in your brain. This is what Suzanne learned to do with her self-hypnosis technique.

Think of it this way: imagine a trail through high grasses in a meadow. As the way is increasingly well established, you will more and more easily tread that path. In our society, most of us have highly activated sympathetic nervous systems, and we move into the stress response with great familiarity. The route that defines the parasympathetic relaxation response is less well worn and more challenging to access. Unless we train ourselves to elicit the relaxation response, it will not come easily to most of us.

Creating a practice that allows you to switch gears serves people well because stress is a part of life, and always has been. Plagues, famine, war, and disruption have always been part of the human experience. In ancient society, after a day of hunting and gathering, our ancestors might light a fire and sit around it long into the night, singing and telling stories. That was their way of reducing stress, but we have mostly lost these habits to modern culture. In Eastern cultures, there has been more emphasis on teaching people how to center and quiet themselves through meditation and breath work. This focus is largely absent in Western society. When I ask people, "What do you do to relax?" they'll often say, "I watch TV," or "I go to the movies," or "I go shopping." These activities can be relaxing, but they don't typically activate the physiological relaxation response. Practices that do activate the relaxation response include breathing exercises, meditation, body scanning, yoga, and tai chi.

Breath Work

Breath work is incredibly beneficial; our breath is free, it is always with us, we can learn techniques quickly, and we may do them anywhere without equipment. It's a physiological fact that you can't be stressed and relaxed at the same time, so breathing is literally a way to change your physiology. Breathing is one of the few things we can do completely consciously or unconsciously because it is controlled by two sets of nerves: the voluntary nervous system and involuntary (autonomic) nervous system. Breathing thus provides a way to gain further control over the involuntary system, and to quiet the nervous system.

Slow, deep breathing is a centerpiece of most mind-body techniques. When you are stressed and can't relax, one strategy you can always use is to slow and deepen your breathing. Often we breathe very shallowly, and expand only the tops of our lungs. One way in which I instruct my patients to do diaphragmatic breathing is as follows: Lie on your back and put a book on your belly. Relax your stomach muscles and inhale deeply so the book rises when you inhale and falls when you exhale. You can see the book rising and falling, which shows that you are bringing air into the lower

129

part of your lungs. Another way to learn diaphragmatic breathing is to sit up straight with your right hand on your belly, left hand on your chest. Breathe in deeply so your right hand rises and falls, and your left hand stays relatively still.

Another breathing exercise involves counting your breaths. You breathe in to a count of one; out to a count of one. Then breathe in to a count of two, out to a count of two, and so on. Think only about the sequential numbers as you breathe in and out. If your mind drifts to a thought (and it will), start over again at one. You can attempt to go up to a count of ten, but it's entirely normal never to get beyond two. If you do get to ten, then go back to one again—it's not a competition; it's breath-focused meditation.

I also teach my patients the 4–7–8 breath, which is a yogic breathing practice that I learned from Dr. Andrew Weil (see the box). It's a superb way to tone the parasympathetic nervous system. I do this breathing exercise twice a day and recommend it to most of the patients who come to the Arizona Center for Integrative Medicine clinic.

4–7–8 Breath (from Pranayama yoga practice)

1. Place the tip of your tongue against the ridge behind and above your front teeth. Keep it there through the whole exercise.
2. Exhale completely through your mouth, making a "whoosh" sound.
3. Inhale deeply and quietly through your nose to a count of four (with mouth closed).
4. Hold your breath for a count of seven.
5. Exhale through your mouth to a count of eight, making a sound.
6. Repeat steps 3, 4, and 5 for a total of four breaths.

You may count slowly or quickly to yourself; what is important is the ratio 4–7–8 rather than the actual speed. Initially some people feel slightly light-headed when learning this breathing technique, but that passes with practice. This exercise can be done in any position; if seated, keep your back straight. I ask my patients to do it regularly, twice daily. It is the regularity of the practice that helps settle the autonomic nervous system. This breathing exercise is remarkable for its simplicity and its brevity. Over the course of just weeks, I have seen this practice lead to significant reduction in anxiety, lowered blood pressure, and greater calm. In addition to your twice-a-day regular practice, you can use it whenever you feel stressed or anxious. While you should not do more than four breath cycles at one time, you can repeat the exercise as often as you wish.

There are literally thousands of different breathing practices in pranayama. One last meditative breathing practice that I love comes from the Vietnamese Buddhist teacher and poet Thich Nhat Hanh. He instructs you to sit quietly and begin to notice your breathing. Then recite in your head, in sync with your inhalation and exhalation:

> Breathing in, I notice my body
> Breathing out, I smile at my body.

Thich Nhat Hanh asks that we make the quality of that smile mirror the quality inherent in a mother smiling at her newborn child. Most of us do not smile at our bodies in this way. Instead we worry about a bit of extra weight here or a wrinkle there. Imagine how your relationship to your body might change if you gave your own body the same love that you intend to give your child.

Meditation

Meditation is another technique for eliciting the relaxation response, and you can do it in many ways. Meditation can focus on the breath, on a mantra, on sounds, or on a candle. Breath counting, as described above, is one example of breath-focused meditation; there are many. Mantras are any words that help you to center yourself; you can use "love," "peace," "om," "beloved child," or a phrase from a prayer from your religious tradition. Again focus your mind on that phrase on the in-breath, and then again on the out-breath. When you notice that your mind has wavered, which it will do repeatedly, you just bring it back. Some people find that using tapes to guide them is the easiest way for them to learn to meditate. A wonderful resource is the Web site www.healthjourneys.com, put together by guided-imagery pioneer Belleruth Naparstek, which offers a wide range of inexpensive CDs to choose from.

Body Scanning

Another way to elicit the relaxation response is by body scanning. In this practice, you lie on your back and focus on your breathing, gently scanning the body and directing breath slowly to each part until all is still. You literally practice moving your mind from your feet to your head, slowly, body part by body part, noticing sensations and directing relaxing breath into each part. You might spend a little extra time on your uterus, noticing as it readies itself to receive a new life.

To start, lie down on your back and take a deep breath. Then begin with the toes of the left foot and slowly move up the foot and leg, feeling the sensations as you go and directing the breath to each area. From the pelvis, move to the toes of the right foot and move up the right leg back to the pelvis. From there, send your breath up through the torso, the lower back and abdomen, the upper back and chest, and the shoulders. Then direct your breath to the fingers of both hands, the wrists, and simultaneously move up both arms, returning to the shoulders. Then send your breath to the neck and throat, and finally the face, back of the head, and the very top of the head.

Now imagine letting your breath move across your entire body from head to foot, as if it were flowing in through the top of the head and out through the toes, and then in through the toes and out through the top of the head.

Sometimes by the end of a body scan, it feels as if the body has dropped away and the breath flows with ease across the entire body. As you complete the scan, enjoy the stillness within.

When you are done, take another deep breath and bring your mind and body back to ordinary consciousness.

Progressive Muscle Relaxation

Progressive muscle relaxation is similar to body scanning. In this practice, you learn to apply tension to groups of muscles, release them, then note how they relax. This serves to heighten your awareness of tensed versus relaxed muscles. Gradually, when you notice yourself "tensing up," you can relax your body, which in turn calms your mind.

Follow the same basic pattern as in body scanning. Lying on your back, start with a deep cleansing breath. Begin by tightly tensing the muscles in both feet, then release the tension. Now sequentially move up your body to each major muscle group, tensing firmly, holding, and then releasing. Move from your calves and thighs, on to your pelvis, your buttocks, abdomen, and shoulder girdle. Then tense the fingers of both hands into tight fists, tightening your forearms and upper arms next. Release them and move to the small muscles in your face. Squint your expression and let it go, move your jaw back and forth, raise your eyebrows and drop them. Lastly, tense your entire body as tightly as you can, and then release.

Herbert Benson's pioneering research affirmed the need for self-care to balance the frenzy in life. Absent today in most of our society is a culture of relaxation. People say, "I'm too busy to relax," or "I don't have time for meditation." But if you understand that your frenzied lifestyle makes your body less receptive to conception, you may become more motivated to take the time to access the relaxation response. Even short practices can have a profound effect on cultivating calm; the power is in their regularity.

Do make a mind-body practice part of your daily routine, because evidence shows that within two to four weeks of a twenty-minute daily meditation or breathing practice, your body begins to benefit from the carryover effect. You may experience lower blood pressure and heart rate; more energy; reduced levels of chemicals in the blood associated with anxiety; and improved immune system function. During this interval, the effect on your nervous system becomes long-lasting. Once it carries over for a full twenty-four hours, you receive prolonged value from the practice, thus quieting your nervous system and helping you to manage whatever stress is present in your life.

Other Stress Management Techniques

While journaling, exercise, and cognitive behavior interventions don't elicit the relaxation response, they do help in managing stress. I will discuss these various methods for helping to balance life; again, choose those that work best for you as an individual.

Cognitive Restructuring

Cognitive restructuring is a behavioral technique that addresses the idea that our thoughts cause our feelings and behaviors. It reveals to us that our stress can be generated from within as well as come from external events. Hence we can change the way we think in order to feel better, even if the situation remains the same. As Alice Domar describes it, our thoughts can determine our emotional states, and our emotional states can influence our physical health. Cognitive restructuring teaches us to remember that our feelings about something are not the same as reality. We have the power to challenge negative thought patterns that circle around in our heads like endlessly repeating audiotapes. Loretta LaRoche, a comedian who teaches mind-body practices, says that you should think of your mind as a bus. Ask yourself, who's driving the bus? It could be your parents, your boss, or anyone else whose past negative messages have gotten stuck in your mind. The goal is to ensure that you are driving your own "bus."

Dr. Domar teaches us to identify when we are having a negative thought by asking ourselves four questions:

1. Does the thought contribute to my stress?
2. Where did I learn this thought (which I may not even truly believe at this point)?
3. Is this thought logical?
4. Is this thought true?

For instance, a patient whom I'll call Leila had been bulimic when she was a young teenager. The bulimia temporarily stopped her periods; once she resumed eating normally, her periods returned. When she was in her late twenties and trying to conceive, Leila believed that she would never be able to get pregnant because of the long-ago effects of her eating disorder.

Together, Leila and I went through Dr. Domar's questions to sort out whether there was any truth in her belief. She admitted that this thought was certainly stressful for her. She realized during our conversation that it had been "planted" by the nutritionist she saw at the time. (She acknowledged that the nutritionist was probably using everything she could think of to get her to change her unhealthy behavior.) Leila was also able to see that the logic was poor, given her current normal menstrual cycles and her healthy cervical mucus. She was happy to conclude that, in answer to question four, the thought was unlikely to be true, and breathed a deep sigh of relief.

Cognitive restructuring has been used to alleviate a wide range of conditions including anxiety, chronic pain, and even arthritis. It helps people to recognize distorted thoughts, "reframe" the situation, and substitute more realistic and positive thoughts and beliefs, which can reduce painful feelings. Here's another example: after a failed trial of Clomid, a woman may engage in "all-or-nothing" thinking, such as, "I'm useless. My body won't ever function like a normal woman's!" Or a person may "catastrophize" a mistake, exaggerate its importance, or jump to unlikely conclusions: "My bus was late this morning, making me late for work. They'll think I'm irresponsible and fire me. Now I won't be able to pay my bills."

Helen Adrienne points out, "Cognitive restructuring can be used to take responsibility for exploring your underlying belief system, rather than suffering with a sense that your infertility is somehow your fault. You have a chance for resolving certain inner conflicts and neutralizing the 'conversation' that the mind and body might be having with one another."

Susan Seeger shared this story about how she freed herself of ambivalence during her attempt to conceive, using cognitive restructuring:

> At thirty-four, I married someone I'd been in a long relationship with. Shortly afterward, we stopped using birth control and attempted to conceive. Ten months later, I had an early miscarriage. While it was agonizing, I recognized the good news, too: that I could get pregnant.
>
> I did all the scientific things, but also treated my spirit. I went to an infertility clinic and went on Clomid, and also went to a psychic, because I thought that if someone saw a baby in my future, I wouldn't mind how long the process took. Still, I had to renew my faith every month when I got my period, and I had to deal with feelings of loss every single night. My husband and I were very much in it together, although I felt as if I cared more than he did because he already had a son from a previous marriage.
>
> We decided to go to Canyon Ranch to spend some time together as a couple, to rest and take a break from the constant disappointment. There we met Devorah Coryell, a grief counselor on staff. We told her that we were struggling with infertility, and she had me lie on the floor of her office and visualize myself as a nineteen-year-old. She took me back in my mind, asking me to

describe what I looked like and where I was. I told her that I was standing in front of the Student Union. Devorah said, "If I run up to you and ask, 'Do you want to have children?' what would you say?" Answering as a nineteen-year-old, I replied, "Not for a really, really long time."

That was the lightbulb moment that got me in touch with my fear. I was the oldest of five children, and my nickname had been "Little Mother." I was my mom's assistant, and a parentified child; I'd had the experience of being a mother when I felt too young for the task. This was a moment of profound insight for me; I understood my infertility. At the deepest level, I was able to let go of my fear.

My husband and I came home, and within a few months, I got pregnant and we had our baby. It was an easy pregnancy and a beautiful birth.

In order to conceive, I had to free up my anxiety, surrender all control, and permit myself to get pregnant. I had to realize that having my own child was different from raising my siblings. I believe that the heart of my infertility was ambivalence; I had the idea of having a baby, but also the fear of having a child. Until I addressed my fears and let the idea of a baby reside inside me, I wasn't going to have one. Since then, I have tried to help other women by telling them about my experience, and my belief about the need to create an environment where a baby would feel welcome.

Cognitive restructuring teaches you to be a witness to your own thoughts as they parade by. I have met women with all sorts of limiting belief systems that were often barely conscious. They varied from fears of being a "bad" mother as a result of the poor mothering they received, to losing their independence or risking their intimacy with their spouses to more superficial fears of the changes pregnancy would bring to their bodies ("My breasts will be ruined; I will get fat; I will no longer be attractive"). Cognitive restructuring can help uncover these buried fears. It teaches us to address the automatic negative thoughts as hypotheses rather than facts. Once these beliefs are exposed, the mind and body can respond differently. And when an appraisal of a situation is accurate, we learn more adaptive ways of responding.

Exercise and Mindful Walking

Another tool that many of us have discovered is exercise. Although it does not directly elicit the relaxation response, oftentimes people find physical activity to be incredibly valuable for managing stress. If I feel anxious about something, exercising vigorously purges the anxiety and moves it out of my physical body and my psyche. I am very grateful that it has that effect on me.

Less vigorous but no less valuable is mindful walking. To walk in this way, pay attention to the sensations in your body. Notice first how your foot touches the ground. Is it the ball or the heel of your foot that hits the ground first? Which muscles tense and which relax? What is the quality of your step like? Then broaden your awareness to take in your surroundings. Listen to the sounds of the birds, feel the air on your skin, or attend to the rise and fall of your chest as you breathe. Notice the world around you. When thoughts come into your mind, and they will, return to the sensations of walking as soon as you become aware that your mind has wandered. A regular practice of mindful walking can be very helpful in relieving stress. In addition, if you're a serious runner and have been told to cut back when you're trying to conceive, mindful walking can be a good way to focus that energy.

Journaling

Journaling is another valuable stress-management tool. You can make it a daily habit to write in a notebook, expressing your thoughts and feelings about your fertility. For some, the act of simply noting your concerns can make them seem more manageable and give you a better handle on stressors in your life. For health benefits, patients are instructed to explore their deepest thoughts and feelings about an experience. They may link it to an experience in childhood, significant relationships, or even their careers. The writing can tie the experience to who you have been in the past, who you would like to be in the future, or who you are now. What is most important is to write honestly and openly for fifteen minutes a day. Occasionally people feel worse when they first start to express their feelings, but this is almost always followed by more positive feelings later. Research shows that writing about stressful events, four days in a row, for fifteen to thirty minutes per day, leads to health benefits, such as reduced long-term stress and disease, that endure for six months. The mechanism by which journaling works is that it allows people to develop coherent stories about events. Expressing facts and feelings with no holds barred helps stop the continued cycle of experiencing and suppressing negative images and memories.

Hypnotherapy

Many people find hypnotherapy helpful in managing stress. When a person is hypnotized, his or her awareness is narrowly focused, fostering a deep sense of relaxation and an openness to posthypnotic suggestions. Also, while hypnotized, people are encouraged to suspend criticism or disbelief—the hallmark of the conscious, thinking mind—and allow trust in the intelligence of the unconscious mind to help them navigate around learned limitations.

Helen Adrienne frequently uses hypnosis with her patients; as she sees it, "Hypnosis speaks the language of the limbic system of the brain, which includes the amygdala. The amygdala holds traumatic memories, and does not respond to 'talk therapy.'" Instead, the hypnotherapist aims to achieve relaxation and comfort, and then reaches the limbic system through indirect approaches such as stories, metaphors, and wordplay. Relief is achieved as the limbic structures accept suggestions to alter one's body chemistry. Hypnosis is also valuable in supporting IVF.

Hypnosis research supports hypnosis's ability to relieve stress-induced infertility. Dr. Sarah Berga led a study of twelve women with functional hypothalamic amenorrhea (stress-induced absence of menstruation). In the study, each woman had one forty-five- to seventy-minute session of hypnotherapy and was then observed for twelve weeks. The women were asked whether menstruation resumed, and about their overall well-being and self-confidence. Nine out of twelve participants got their periods, and all twelve women described improvement in general well-being and overall self-confidence. While this was a small study, it is remarkable that one hypnotherapy session resulted in resumption of menstruation in 75 percent of the women, and in a broad positive effect in all.

Can Stress Reduction Enhance Fertility?

While stress may be implicated in infertility, learning that you are having difficulty with conception—or worse, being labeled infertile—raises stress levels even more. Infertility is so incredibly stressful that it has been shown to be on par with HIV or cancer. One survey looked at 121 couples dealing with infertility; 19 percent of the women experienced moderate depression; 13 percent had severe depression; and 26 percent were at high risk for sexual dysfunction. Many, but not all, studies have found that depressive symptoms may decrease the success rate of fertility treatment. But can stress reduction relieve infertility? The answer appears to be a tentative yes.

Dr. Alice Domar used a mind-body skills-building course with 184 women who were experiencing infertility. Most had been trying to conceive for one to two years, and all were under the care of reproductive endocrinologists. Initially Dr. Domar wanted to see if she could help the women cope with the incredible stress they were experiencing. To her delight and surprise, she found that the group learned to cope with the stress and had higher pregnancy rates as well.

Dr. Domar has gone on to train therapists around the world to lead mind-body groups, and some have replicated her research. They have found that mind-body interventions can help people cope with depression and anxiety, and may improve levels of optimism. And a few of these studies, like Dr. Domar's, suggest that mind-body programs enhance fertility.

Researcher Dr. Jacky Boivin did a meta-analysis of psychological interventions for infertility, looking at pregnancy rates, psychological distress (including anxiety and depression), and interpersonal functioning. The meta-analysis revealed that educational programs were more effective than counseling, and that the best type of mind-body program for infertility is one that teaches stress management, relaxation, and coping skills. She also found that mind-body support groups work better than individual therapy. Some of us are shy or private, and prefer not to share personal matters in public. Infertility is often kept secret, which can make us feel isolated. These studies suggest, however, that the peer support gained from the group experience may be worth someone's departing from her comfort zone. A second meta-analysis showed that a minimum of six sessions of cognitive behavioral therapy, relaxation training, bad-health-habit modification, and social support is more effective than fewer sessions; in other words, like any new habit, it takes time to accrue the benefits of these new practices.

Helen Adrienne has been conducting mind-body stress-reduction groups for many years. She believes the groups provide coping skills that serve people throughout their lives by improving their ability to handle any kind of adversity. Her patients describe that they feel back in control—not of being infertile, but in how they handle the infertility.

The Effects of Infertility and Miscarriage

Infertility represents the loss of a dream, and in a way it is experienced as a death. As Helen Adrienne puts it, "We are born, we grow up, reproduce, and die; reproduction is germane to our existence. When you can't conceive, it's as if the universe is saying 'no' to you."

A recent study analyzed the experience of nineteen Israeli women who lost their first pregnancies to miscarriage but later went on to have children. The miscarriages undermined the women's basic belief in their fertility, as well as threatened their sense of the meaning of life and their roles as women. Of these women, 70 percent reported anxiety, difficulty falling asleep, helplessness, and repeated recollection of the experience. In addition, the loss of the first pregnancy led the women to question their future ability to have children and their self-image as mothers. The women felt that it was difficult to get the support they needed; even when someone said she understood, they didn't believe it unless the person had gone through a miscarriage herself. Similarly, they felt that their husbands did not completely understand what they were going through. On the other hand, talking to their own mothers was found to be very helpful.

Marriage and Partnership

Often, men and women deal with the challenges of infertility and miscarriage in widely varying manners. Adrienne says, "For both men and women, infertility is   141 a bio-psycho-socio-spiritual crisis. But the sexes tend to experience infertility and miscarriage very differently." Men may want to fix things; women often need to feel them. Many men aren't brought up with the emotional experience to be involved in this challenge, and they may not know how to react to someone so distraught. Some men are taught not to honor their own feelings; it's a death for men as well, but some need to learn to feel and express it in order to be fully present to their partners. Every once in a while a couple reverses these typical roles, but Adrienne says that no matter who is in what role, the challenge is an opportunity to build greater intimacy.

In contrast, some couples found that struggling with fertility actually strengthened their marriages. In one large study, two-thirds of the couples reported benefits. These couples related that they were forced to discuss the emotional aspects of infertility as well as existential aspects of life. They learned to manage new, stressful situations together, thereby improving their mutual connection. The researchers found that couples typically used one of four strategies to cope with childlessness: (1) active-avoidance strategies (e.g., avoiding being with pregnant women or children); (2) active-confronting strategies (e.g., showing feelings, asking others for advice, and talking with other people about emotional aspects of infertility); (3) passive-avoidance strategies (e.g., hoping for a miracle); and (4) meaning-based coping (e.g., thinking about the fertility problem in a positive light, and finding other goals in life). Active-confronting coping was a significant predictor of high marital benefit for men, while an active-avoidance strategy predicted the opposite. In women, those who used meaning-based coping strategies experienced reduced distress. Knowing that one strategy tends to be more effective than another can help shape our behavior when faced with infertility.

Is This in Any Way My Fault?

One challenge inherent in teaching people about mind-body therapies is an implied blame. The logic is as follows: if I can use my mind to help me heal, did I cause the problem to begin with? I always address this. While I routinely recommend mind-body strategies, I tell my patients that diseases are multi-factorial—with genetic, environmental, lifestyle, infectious, and traumatic origins.

When I asked Dr. Domar about how she frames the mind-body relationship to women, she said, "When we speak about stress, it implies that the patient is to blame. The body is very wise; there is an ancient part of the brain that we carry with us, and if our body doesn't feel that the time is ideal to conceive, the ancient part of the brain won't let you. In the time of the caveman, if a woman was experiencing stress, it meant that environmental conditions were not optimal for conception, and that carries through to the modern day. Your body doesn't know you're stressed because your boss is a jerk; it thinks you are being chased by a saber-toothed tiger. Women have to realize that being stressed and having trouble getting pregnant is not their fault."

Helen Adrienne says, "If we suggest that people can do better by using the mind-body connection, there is an inherent sense of blame; in other words, you don't handle stress well. There is a subterranean rumble; people sense this and blame themselves. You are not responsible for your fertility, but you can be responsible *to* it. You can control your response to your environment, even though you can't control the environment itself."

If fertility is being impacted by the mind-body connection, it is likely coming from an unconscious place. Yet if you bring the problem to your conscious awareness, you may be able to work through it. Many women have underlying fears that they have never dealt with; uncovering these long-buried issues can at times reverse their effects. For example, a woman who has had bad mothering can be afraid of becoming her own mother. There is the fear of pregnancy, the fear of having a girl when the husband really wants a son, and the fear of giving birth. If you can get to the bottom of the fear, you may find that you are released from it.

A patient of mine who had a son after several years of infertility told me that the struggle to have a child "really defines us as parents—it makes us so appreciative. I wouldn't trade the experience of our really challenging introduction to parenthood, because it led me to be the mother I am today." Another woman told me that the challenges eventually made her more present as a mother, and brought out her strength.

143

The Three A's, as Taught by Helen Adrienne

Acceptance (because nothing can change without acceptance of what is)

Awareness (of who you and your partner are, as well as the people in your family and your world)

Adaptation (using mind-body techniques so you don't feel so out of control; thus you can be in control of the way in which you journey toward conception)

In closing this chapter, I want to share some of my own mind-body practices. You may be surprised at how many I do. For my daily practice, I do the 4–7–8 breath twice a day. I also "breathe" before answering the phone and take a deep diaphragmatic breath to clear myself before I go in to see a patient.

In addition, I have several weekly practices. I have practiced hatha yoga once or twice a week for almost twenty years. I have a very busy mind, and it's often difficult for me to quiet my thoughts. Toward the middle of a yoga class, I find that my mind has quieted and I'm very focused on my breath and on the asana practice. At the end of class, when I lie on the floor in savasana, or corpse pose, I feel a profound sense of relaxation. I always notice how yoga leaves me centered, with a relaxed mind; it also leaves me feeling really happy.

I'm lucky to have a labyrinth on my land near Tucson that I walk regularly as a meditative practice. I spend time looking at the beauty of nature, which I find very powerful. I am blessed to live in a place with gorgeous mesquite trees and wildflowers, a view of the mountains, and many birds, bunnies, and prairie dogs circling around. Maintaining an awareness of the beauty of nature is powerful for me. On weekends, I take a seven-mile sunset hike in Sabino Canyon. Watching the light change on the mountains and being in a place that I have grown to love is centering; my connection to nature is part of my spiritual practice that has a far-reaching impact on me.

Finally, I attempt to go off on a retreat once or twice a year. The power of taking a complete break from my regular busy schedule has a profound effect that goes far beyond the time spent away. This serves as a restorative practice that helps me recenter, think about my priorities, and reflect upon how well I am living my life in accord with those priorities.

Consider the ways that you can incorporate mind-body practices in your own life. While I can make suggestions, it's better for you to select the strategies that will work best in your life. Can you go for a mindful walk three days a week? Write in a journal before you go to bed? Do you have time for a yoga class? I recommend that everyone do simple breath work twice a day. Begin with the things that resonate, are easiest to include in your schedule, or most intrigue you. It's okay to experiment until you settle in to those that you want to turn into regular practices. The benefits of mind-body work are far-reaching, and will help you feel more serene and relaxed about your fertility quest.

CHAPTER 7

CONVENTIONAL MEDICINE

Before You Conceive

While having a baby is one of the most "natural" things in the world, a visit to the doctor may still be in order. It is true that there are many things we can do to enhance the likelihood of having healthy children. Whether it is ensuring that you are immune to measles and chicken pox, taking a multivitamin with folic acid, or stopping a contraindicated medication or an environmental exposure, there is much to review in a preconception visit with your physician.

As an integrative physician, I regularly use the many advances available in conventional medicine. I am deeply appreciative of all that it has to offer to promote good health before conception, to assess fertility problems, and to treat infertility when necessary. Conventional medicine can be simply miraculous, allowing women and men who previously wouldn't have been able to conceive to bear children.

I highly recommend that when a woman first starts thinking about getting pregnant, she meet with her doctor. Dr. Carl Sgarlata is a reproductive endocrinologist based in the Bay Area. He, too, counsels patients to get into the best possible health before conception, so that they are more in control of their own fertility. In addition to multivitamins with folic acid for women, he recommends an antioxidant formula for men, since increased antioxidants aid sperm morphology, or normal structure. If the patient has not already used an ovulation predictor kit, he may ask her to use one for a couple of months to check ovulatory timing.

Dr. Sgarlata finds that many patients come to him with incomplete prior care. Of the women that he sees, 25 percent are not taking folic acid; others have not been screened for rubella or chicken pox. In addition, many people have not received appropriate genetic counseling for cystic fibrosis, thalassemia, or Tay-Sachs. He has also seen women who were treated with Clomid before their male partners had semen analyses—which is putting the cart before the horse when you consider that male factors are responsible for up to 40 percent of infertility.

Dr. Sgarlata states that while he is not convinced that stress alone causes infertility, he does believe that stress *influences* fertility. He asks his patients how they manage the stress of day-to-day living, and what tools they have to help manage worry and anxiety. He feels that patients need to understand the importance of mind-body practices, and be motivated to make lifestyle changes.

While some women are nervous about going to the doctor, it is important to make sure you are in the best possible health before trying to conceive. I describe what to expect at your preconception visit below.

Overall Health

Your overall well-being is of vital importance, and addressing health issues before pregnancy is the ideal. If you are overweight, I would advise you to lose weight in order to conceive more easily, reduce the risk of gestational diabetes, and improve the health of your baby. I would discuss lifestyle issues such as smoking, exercise, alcohol consumption, and other topics. Even your dental health matters: gum disease due to bacteria can be transmitted to your baby, increasing the risk of preterm labor as well as childhood cavities and poor dental health. Getting your blood pressure or diabetes under excellent control (or even better, reversing them with lifestyle changes) is a worthwhile endeavor before conceiving a new life.

Vitamins and Medications

While it is recommended that all women of childbearing age take multivitamins with folic acid to help prevent neural tube defects in their babies, 67 percent of young women are not taking such a vitamin. Certain medications such as Accutane, prescribed for acne, are contraindicated during pregnancy, and should be stopped. Other medicines must be at exactly the right dose to assure fertility, thyroid-replacement medicine being one example.

Men may be taking medicines that affect sperm; for example, calcium channel blockers, a class of blood pressure medication, interfere with the sperm's ability to penetrate the egg. Spironolactone, another antihypertensive, can impair production of testosterone and sperm. Medicines used to treat colitis, such as sulfasalazine, affect normal sperm development, as can the antibiotics tetracycline, gentamicin, and erythromycin. In most cases, an alternative medication can be prescribed when a couple is thinking about getting pregnant.

Also during this visit, your doctor can explore possible environmental exposures; for example, if you are a nurse working in a hospital, bisphenol A is ubiquitous—and an endocrine disruptor; you should also avoid hand cleansers with triclosan, chemotherapeutic agents, and bringing people in for radiation therapy. If you work in an environment where chemicals are frequently used, such as a dry cleaner, printing company, pharmaceutical lab, factory, or agricultural locale, you may need to alter your work duties. Other environmental exposures, such as the artificial hormones in meat and the carcinogenic chemicals in sunscreen, and a range of nutritional choices are worth considering when preparing to make yourself a welcoming host for new life.

Basic Lab Work

Basic lab work is advised as well. This includes blood tests to check for immunity to German measles (rubella) and chicken pox. If you are not immune, there is time to get vaccinated before pregnancy. Other labs that I suggest assess for anemia, suboptimal thyroid function, and vitamin D levels.

Your doctor may also discuss what to expect in terms of the likelihood of conception. Although 85 percent of couples do get pregnant within six to eight months of

149

unprotected midcycle intercourse, some couples believe that they will conceive right away and are surprised when it takes longer than they had anticipated.

In these discussions, your doctor may pick up on potential warning signs that could signal future difficulty conceiving. For example, I saw a lovely, twenty-six-year-old woman whom I'll call Marie. She said that she had had very rare periods over the past year, and prior to that, perhaps eight or nine periods per year. Normally a thin person, she had experienced an unusual weight gain of 30 pounds; she was constipated and fatigued, her skin was dry, and her mood, depressed. Her physical exam was normal except that her thyroid gland was slightly enlarged. Marie told me that she had tried diet and increased exercise, but to no avail. Her primary care doctor had run labs for her: she was not anemic and had a normal thyroid and thyroid-stimulating hormone (TSH). Her doctor told her that she was worrying too much and needed to exercise more.

Marie felt as if she had tried everything to lose weight and feel better, but that nothing had worked. As I listened to Marie's description of her symptoms, they sounded like classic hypothyroidism. Even though her lab tests were normal, I prescribed a trial of low-dose thyroid medicine, closely following her thyroid and TSH blood work to make sure she wasn't overtreated. Within six months, her periods normalized and she had a cycle every twenty-nine days. Over the course of one year, she took off all the excess weight, her constipation resolved, her thyroid gland shrank, and her mood lifted. Marie had clinical hypothyroidism yet had normal lab values. While treating a patient with a "normal TSH" is controversial, overreliance on lab tests without attending to the patient's clinical picture can lead to missed diagnoses and inadequate treatment.

I inquire in detail about menstrual cycles, asking my patient how often they occur, their duration, whether she can tell when she is ovulating, and if her luteal phase is short. This is also when I examine for possible signs of PCOS such as excessive facial or body hair, acne, and irregular periods.

Difficulty Conceiving

Although most couples will become pregnant within a year, some will struggle; difficulty conceiving affects approximately one in seven couples. It is usually suggested that further evaluation occur after one year of trying in women under the age of thirty-five; six months in women aged thirty-five to forty; and three months in women over the age of forty. You will notice the paradox here, since the older a woman is, the longer it will take for her to conceive; yet the older she is, the more urgency exists.

If you belong to the 15 percent or so of couples who struggle to conceive, your physicians will want to examine both of you for a variety of conditions. While the percentages vary a bit according to the study reviewed, it is thought that infertility is due to male factors in one-third of all cases, female factors in one-third, and combined male-female factors in the last third.

Fertility Problems in Men

As your physician investigates the reasons that pregnancy is not occurring with ease, it is important to assess the male partner early. A sperm sample is easy to obtain, and much less invasive compared to some of the testing that women endure. The semen analysis looks for abnormal sperm production or function. This can be due to a wide range of causes, from an undescended testicle, to genetic disease such as cystic fibrosis, to environmental exposures or a history of cancer with radiation or chemotherapeutic treatment. Infections can lead to a blocked tube. Even lifestyle habits can impact fertility in men: hot tubs, saunas, daily hot baths, or frequent use of laptop computers (on one's lap) can overheat the testes, effectively killing sperm. Poor nutrition, obesity, cigarette smoking, and alcohol use are further culprits. Marked advances have been made for treating male infertility, ranging from antioxidant treatment to ultrasound exploration and needle removal of single sperm cells to be used for intracytoplasmic sperm injections (ICSI) accompanying IVF.

Fertility Problems in Women

When pregnancy has not occurred with ease, investigations can determine if a woman is ovulating, whether she has normal hormone levels, if there is any sign of an infec-

151

tion, whether her fallopian tubes are open, and lastly whether there are any other compromising factors.

The first question that we usually consider is, are you ovulating? One clear indicator that a woman is ovulating is the presence of regular menstrual cycles. As discussed in Chapter 2, "Your Body, Your Lifestyle, and Fertility," to determine whether you are ovulating, you can check your basal body temperature (BBT) or use an ovulation predictor kit. Your doctor can assess ovulation by taking a small amount of cervical mucus and putting it under a microscope. Cervical mucus fans out in a beautiful fern-like pattern at ovulation. At other times of the month, it looks more like random splotches. Finally, most ob-gyns have an ultrasound in their office, and they can use it to check your ovaries for developing follicles.

Your doctor might also check your ovarian reserve. This involves a blood test to measure your FSH level on day 3 of your cycle (day 1 is the first day of your period). The higher your FSH is, the harder your pituitary gland has to work to stimulate your ovaries. In this way, FSH serves as an indirect measure of egg quality; less than 10 is normal, meaning that your ovaries are most likely producing fertilizable eggs. An FSH of 10 to 13 is borderline—it takes a "louder" FSH message to cause an egg to be released. An FSH of over 13 is of concern (yet some women do get pregnant with an FSH of 13 or more). Whenever I see abnormal or borderline labs, I repeat the blood test, just to make sure it was neither a lab error nor an anomaly. Elevated FSH levels are one reason that ovulation-inducing medication or IVF is recommended.

Two more tests for ovarian reserve are worth mentioning. Measuring anti-Mullerian hormone, or AMH, is a newer blood test that can be conducted at any point in the cycle; unlike FSH and estradiol levels, it can even be measured when women are on the birth control pill. AMH is produced by the antral follicles (follicles that appear early in the menstrual cycle, and which indicate how many eggs a woman has). AMH is a better measure of ovarian reserve than FSH, but the test is not always covered by insurance. If AMH is low, IVF with donor eggs might be recommended. Lastly, a vaginal ultrasound on day 3 of your cycle can be used to measure the overall ovarian volume and the number of antral follicles.

Hormone levels are also used to diagnose fertility problems. Unfortunately, hormones such as progesterone, estradiol, and prolactin fluctuate quite a bit, and therefore can be hard to interpret. Dr. Barbi Phelps-Sandall, an integrative ob-gyn in the San Francisco area who graduated from our fellowship program, never checks estradiol. In her opinion, it fluctuates so much that she doesn't find it a helpful barometer. Some doctors check progesterone levels seven days after ovulation, and this provides a retrospective reassurance that you have indeed ovulated—yet progesterone can also fluctuate. Occasionally a doctor will check levels of prolactin, which is the hormone that instructs the breasts to produce milk in nursing mothers; it also suppresses ovulation so that you don't immediately have another baby. If prolactin is elevated, it can interfere with ovulation. In addition, your doctor will check your thyroid levels if that has not already been done.

Dr. Sgarlata points out that some women have very elevated estradiol levels on the second or third day of their cycles, yet their FSH is normal. (Normally estradiol is lowest on days 2 through 5; after that, the follicle begins producing high levels.) If estradiol is elevated early in the cycle, this may suppress the FSH level, giving false reassurance that ovarian reserve is normal. With issues such as hirsutism (unwanted hair growth), he checks androgen levels. If a woman has PCOS, he obtains fasting glucose and insulin levels to look at glucose metabolism; as a result, he may suggest lifestyle or dietary adjustments. Typically he does not do progesterone testing, as he feels that it is hard to say what a normal progesterone level in the luteal phase is, given the wide daily variation in secretion by the corpus luteum.

Other lab work might also be useful. I would consider celiac testing if there is a history of abdominal pain or abnormal bowel movements. Sometimes celiac disease presents in subtle ways, causing skin rashes or joint achiness, so I may order testing even when there are no GI symptoms. Insulin levels and blood sugars are important if PCOS is suspected. Finally, you may be tested for MTHFR (methylenetetrahydrofolate reductase), a genetic variant present in one of ten people of European descent. This variant increases the risk of Down syndrome, miscarriages, and neural tube defects. Men can have it as well, in which case it leads to low sperm counts. MTHFR can be treated effectively with extra folic acid or 1-methyl-folate.

Also explored in the checkup is whether there are any signs of infection in you or your partner. Your physician will take a cervical culture, and will need to treat both partners simultaneously if either of you are infected. Gonorrhea is usually symptom-

153

atic, but chlamydia is generally asymptomatic; in the United States, 409 people per 100,000 are infected. Less common are ureaplasma and mycobacteria. Often these infections cause no symptoms, but they may interfere with fertility. When men have any symptoms at all, it is usually a low-grade urethritis, which is inflammation of the urinary tract that causes burning with urination. Dr. Phelps-Sandell suspects ureaplasma and mycobacteria when a woman has had multiple miscarriages. To treat these infections, a course of antibiotics is prescribed to both partners simultaneously.

The final area that a doctor often checks is whether the woman's fallopian tubes are open and whether there is uterine scarring. She may order a hysterosalpingogram, in which dye is injected into the uterine cavity, or else a sonohystogram, in which the uterine cavity is distended with saline. A laparoscopy, where a small incision is made in the abdomen to introduce a small scope, is done when endometriosis or adhesive disease is suspected.

Infertility

Sometimes, a couple will have done all that they can, been assessed with the lab tests above, adjusted their diet and exercise, begun stress-reduction practices . . . and still have not become pregnant. This is usually due to ovulatory infertility, and here is where the advances in conventional medicine can make all the difference. Ask your ob-gyn how much infertility work she does. If it is not a regular part of her practice, ask for a referral to a reproductive endocrinologist.

Some ob-gyns do more infertility work than others. A common first intervention for infertility is the use of an ovulation inducer. Clomid has been available since the seventies and remains a first choice. If ineffective, injections of FSH and LH may be used. Dr. Phelps-Sandall prescribes low doses of Clomid in order to reduce the risk of multiple pregnancies; she also does a follicle scan on day 12–13 using ultrasound, so that if too many follicles are developing, she can ask the couple to abstain from sexual intercourse in order to avoid a multiple pregnancy. Dr. Phelps-Sandall also offers intrauterine insemination in her office.

For unexplained infertility, Dr. Sgarlata prescribes Clomid along with artificial insemination for a three-cycle trial. While neither the medication nor insemination alone drastically improves the pregnancy rate, combining the two does improve chances of conception. Clomid drives the ovaries to produce more eggs; it may also organize follicular development. Intrauterine insemination (IUI) ensures that the sperm enter the uterus. With sexual intercourse, millions of sperm are deposited in the vagina; ten thousand may make it to the cervix, but only a thousand or so get to the fallopian tube. An IUI increases the odds of fertilization by increasing the number of sperm that arrive near the egg at the appropriate moment.

If the combination of Clomid and artificial insemination doesn't work, substituting injectable FSH and LH for Clomid may be used next. However, more often, if Clomid fails, then Dr. Sgarlata suggests his patient undergo IVF, thereby superseding the challenge of an egg and sperm that are not uniting. The 2010 FASTT Study revealed that going directly to IVF after using Clomid for three cycles (rather than injectable ovulation inducers) led couples to conceive more quickly and with lower cost. Dr. Sgarlata also recommends acupuncture in conjunction with IVF, as he feels that it aids in the transfer and also helps his patients manage stress.

In 2010, the Nobel Prize in Medicine was awarded to Robert Edwards for developing human IVF therapy. His research radically improved medical treatment of infertility, which affects 10 percent of couples worldwide. Since 1978, when Louise Brown, the first "test tube" baby, was born, four million people have been born through IVF. Many are adults now, and are in fact having children of their own.

While IVF is miraculous, it is not risk-free. Ovarian hyperstimulation; multiple births (which are associated with risks such as prematurity and maternal diabetes); long-term bed rest during pregnancy, which causes bone loss and osteoporosis; and premature births all are associated with IVF, as is the concern about slightly increasing the risk of ovarian cancer later in the mother's life. In addition, there can be consequences of immaturity to the baby, as well as higher risks of cerebral palsy and other birth defects in multiple pregnancies.

A recent study from Finland found an increased risk of birth defects in babies conceived from IVF. There were two comparison groups along with the IVF group: naturally conceived babies from the general population and babies who were conceived with non-IVF fertility treatments. The rate of birth defects in the IVF babies was 4.3 percent; the non-IVF fertility treatment rate was 3.7 percent; and the general population rate was 2.9 percent.

For women age forty-two or above, Dr. Sgarlata does not use Clomid, because the live birth rate is only 1 percent. Instead, he goes right to injectable FSH. He points out that in general, IVF pregnancy rates are not high after age forty-two, and he recommends the use of donor eggs to women between the ages of forty-three and forty-five. His IVF program's age cutoff is forty-four if they are using the woman's own eggs, with the caveat that she must have a normal FSH and AMH.

Dr. Sgarlata follows integrative medicine principles, advising three months of traditional Chinese medicine herbal remedies and acupuncture prior to IVF, as well as acupuncture at the time of transfer. He stresses the importance of lifestyle factors, citing a recent study that showed if a woman had four drinks per week, there was a 16 percent reduction in the pregnancy rate. If both members of the couple had four or more drinks per week, the rate dropped by 21 percent.

Media messages commonly imply that women can have children at any age with just a little help from conventional medicine. Rarely is it made clear that one's odds of getting pregnant, even with IVF, are much reduced after age thirty-five. Centers for Disease Control (CDC) statistics show that overall IVF below the age of thirty-five has a 45 percent success rate; between the ages of thirty-five and thirty-seven, it is 37.3 percent effective; between thirty-eight and forty, it is 26.6 percent; between forty-one and forty-two, it is 15.2 percent; and between forty-three and forty-four, it is 6.7 percent. Patients who are in their midthirties and who are not sure when to start families, or whether they want more children, should realize that fertility is not necessarily forgiving if they wait too long.

Two Important Decisions About IVF

While your doctor will need to make many decisions about ovulation induction and IVF, such as dosing and the combination and selection of drugs, there are two very important issues I want you to consider. The first is how many embryos you will want to transfer. It is important to have thought this through with care, so that you have made a decision before the emotional time of transfer—where you're told, for example, that there are five good embryos. At that moment, you are in a heightened emotional state, and it is a bad time to be making major decisions.

We know that multiple births present risks to both the mother and the babies. The risks to the mom include miscarriage, hemorrhage, pregnancy-induced high blood pressure, preeclampsia, gestational diabetes, anemia, polyhydramnios (extra amniotic fluid), C-section, and prolonged hospitalization with greater costs. For the babies, there is a higher risk of preterm delivery (50 to 60 percent for twins, and 90 percent for triplets). The proportion of twins who are delivered before thirty weeks (i.e., severely premature) is 7 percent, and 15 percent for triplets. These babies are more likely to suffer lifelong serious health problems, including cerebral palsy and mental, physical, learning, and behavioral disabilities; there is an eight times higher risk of disability in twins, forty-seven times higher in triplets. Multiple pregnancies have a fourfold increase in the rate of low birth weight compared to single births, and the risk of lifelong disability is over 25 percent if an infant weighs less than 1 kilogram or 2.2 pounds. In addition, there is a higher rate of stillbirths and neonatal deaths in multiple pregnancies compared to singles. With a single birth, the risk of stillbirth or neonatal death is less than 1 percent; with twins, it is 4.7 percent; and for triplets, 8.3 percent. Overall birth defects are twice as common as in single births. In the media, we see images of beautiful twins and triplets, but we don't often hear about the health problems.

Recognizing the above risks, over time, the American Society for Reproductive Medicine has moved toward recommending that fewer and fewer embryos be transferred (depending on maternal age, and allowing more as age increases). As a result, there are fewer multiple births in the United States than previously. In Europe, it is recommended that only one embryo be transferred; of course, this is an easier decision when one has free health care. And I recognize that often a couple feels, it's so difficult to get pregnant, "Let's have our whole family all at once"—still, we do need to consider the risks.

The second important decision is how many times to attempt IVF. With the initial IVF, the live birth rate is 36 percent; 48 percent on the second attempt; and 53 percent on the third. From that point on, the success rate doesn't go up very much.

For women who tried seven or more cycles of IVF, the live birth rate was 56 percent. Therefore it may make sense to limit your number of attempts at IVF to three.

If you make this decision up front, it will also shift your commitment to preparation. While you may want to go right to IVF, because you want a baby so badly, if you knew you were going to give it a maximum of three attempts, you might be more motivated to prepare yourself mentally and physically. I believe that you will increase your odds of having a successful IVF if first you improve your diet, better manage your stress, and have regular acupuncture.

Freezing Eggs

Egg freezing is the newest high-tech recommendation for women to beat their biological clocks. Women in their early thirties are being offered the chance to freeze their eggs if they are not currently in relationships but want children eventually. However, as of 2012, egg freezing is still considered experimental by the American Society for Reproductive Medicine. To date, there have been only approximately five thousand live births as a result of egg freezing. Often Dr. Sgarlata sees patients aged thirty-eight to forty-five who want to freeze their eggs; he considers this to be too late. In the latter thirties and the forties, ovarian stimulation does not produce as many eggs, and they are not as viable as those of younger women.

There are a number of problems involved in egg freezing that women should consider. Oocytes, the female reproductive cells, are the largest cells in the body, and until recently, have been very difficult to freeze due to the large amount of cytoplasm (fluid) in the cell. A new technique, called vitrification, which flash freezes the cell, has improved the success rates. To undergo egg freezing, a woman must have her ovaries hyperstimulated with medications and undergo a small surgical procedure for retrieval, just as if she were doing an IVF. Not many eggs are produced with each cycle—perhaps ten to twenty—so that the woman must go through several cycles in order to bank a reasonable number of eggs.

Egg freezing does allow for the preservation of eggs in younger women who have normal FSH levels. Pregnancy rates through egg freezing have improved to 30 percent when the eggs are frozen, thawed at a later date, inseminated, and placed in the woman's body.

At present, most egg freezing is provided to women who have cancer diagnoses, when the chemo or radiation therapy will affect their fertility. Another investigational technique used for these women is taking a small section of ovary and freezing it. After treatment, the ovary can be reimplanted in the woman's body, or the eggs can be coaxed to mature in the lab. Another conventional approach, if a woman is having only radiation therapy, is to use ovarian transposition, where the ovary is moved away from the pelvis and into the abdominal cavity, and thus protected from the radiation.

Dr. Sgarlata states that in his experience, most women do not proceed with egg freezing once they realize all that is involved. You have to ask yourself to what extent you are willing to place yourself at a health risk in order to potentially get pregnant at some future moment, particularly since it is not known how long eggs can be frozen and successfully thawed.

Infertility can be baffling and complex, and can lead to pain and suffering. Often, in every other aspect of women's lives, they are able to attain anything they truly desire. Whether it is an education, a job, or a new car, resourceful women find ways to achieve their goals. It can be exceedingly difficult to come to terms with the reality that conception is not entirely under one's control.

CHAPTER 8

TRADITIONAL CHINESE MEDICINE

One of my teachers, Dr. Qingcai Zhang, taught me that traditional Chinese medicine (TCM) holds that the entire purpose of medicine is "to dispel evil and support the good." In Western medicine, the primary focus is almost entirely upon dispelling evil. Think about many of our medications: we have antibiotics (to remove bacteria from the body), antihistamines (to stop the release of histamine produced by contact with an allergen), and anti-hypertensives (to counteract high blood pressure).

Chinese medicine, on the other hand, reminds us that we need to support the good. It does this through a wide range of recommendations and treatments, including dietary change, meditation, qi gong, acupuncture, herbs, *tui na* (massage), and moxibustion (bringing heat to the meridians). Rather than attacking bacteria or depressing the blood pressure, the goal is to bring a person's body back into harmony so that it can heal its own physical challenges.

Much of this book is about supporting the good—preparing body, mind, and spirit to become a container for new life. Using a gardening metaphor, consider all that is needed to grow healthy plants. The soil needs attention; it must be neither too wet nor too dry. It needs the right balance of nitrogen and other fertilizers. Mulching is indicated at times, as is knowing how much and when to prune. Plant a seed too early, and it may be killed by frost; too late, and it may miss the growing season.

The gardening metaphor is often used to describe the way in which TCM seeks to bring harmony and balance to the body; this is applicable to our understanding of fertility as we seek to help women achieve balance in their lives, to ensure ease in conception and healthy pregnancies. TCM philosophy has broadly influenced that of integrative medicine. While Western medicine does take note of the concept of balance, in its recognition of the body's maintenance of homeostasis, it is much less emphasized, and there are fewer tools and practices to help attain balance than there are in Chinese medicine.

I have long been fascinated by traditional Chinese medicine, which began more than two thousand years ago. As executive director of the Arizona Center for Integrative Medicine for more than a decade, I have attended weekly patient conferences that include TCM practitioners, naturopathic doctors, osteopaths, nutritionists, pharmacists, homeopaths, shamans, and energy healers as well as Western-trained physicians. Over the course of many years participating in this dialogue about patients and their medical problems, I have absorbed the worldviews of the different approaches to health and healing. Chinese medicine fascinates me with its theories about how we are connected with natural cycles of the earth, the seasons, and lunar cycles. It seems that every aspect of the natural world and its relation to human beings has been considered, which makes TCM unbelievably rich and complex.

Over the years, I have referred many patients to TCM. Sometimes they use it as primary treatment, as in the cases of women who desire to avoid hormones and need help with menopausal symptoms; other times it serves as an adjunct, such as for women undergoing chemotherapy. My patients often describe the benefit in general terms. They experience enhanced energy and an improved sense of well-being. For women with fertility challenges, they notice more regular periods, a change in the quality of the menstrual blood itself, more abundant cervical mucus, and most important, a greater ease conceiving and carrying their children to term.

My patients' experiences prompted me to investigate whether there are common TCM diagnoses in women labeled by Western doctors as infertile. An Australian study of 180 women examined this very question, considering women who underwent assisted reproductive technology as well as a traditional Chinese medicine evaluation. The researchers found that the most common TCM diagnosis was kidney yang deficiency, which affected 54 percent of the women in the study. Certain conditions were linked; for example, the TCM diagnosis of either qi or blood stagnation was associated with poorer quality of life in the mental-health or social-function domain. As research continues in this area, it will be fascinating to find the commonalties and differences between Western and Chinese medical thought.

TCM theory includes several core beliefs, including essence; yin and yang; and the three vital substances. *Essence* is the body's properties that are present at birth; *yin and yang* is the theory of balancing opposites; the *three vital substances* are qi and blood, along with essence. TCM also holds specific theories about the menstrual cycle, stress, and the movement of the vital substances. In this section, I will describe each of these aspects of TCM theory.

TCM Theory

1. Essence: the body's properties that are present at birth.
2. Yin and yang: the theory of balancing opposites.
3. The three vital substances: qi, blood, and essence.

Essence

Essence is inherited by each individual at birth and matures in seven-year intervals. At age fourteen (2 x 7), there is the arrival of a woman's period, called the "heavenly waters." The menstrual cycle is the expression of abundance of essence and blood; it gathers every twenty-eight days with the lunar cycle. The abundance of essence peaks at age twenty-eight (another factor of seven), and this is considered the ideal time

163

to have a child; then at thirty-five, essence and fertility begin to decline. At 7 x 7, or forty-nine, a woman's essence is dramatically reduced, ending her ability to conceive. It's interesting to me how closely aligned Chinese medicine is to Western medicine with respect to the influence of one's age upon fertility.

Yin and Yang

Chinese medicine is based in the theory of yin and yang, or the balance of opposites. Yin is equated with substance, stillness, moisture, darkness, the interior, and coolness. Yang includes energy, metabolic processes, transformation, heat, the exterior, brightness, activity, and dryness. As Leslie McGee, a nurse and a diplomate in acupuncture and Chinese herbology, describes it, "Yin and yang are opposites, and can consume one another. For example, yin's moisture can extinguish yang's heat, while yang's heat can dry yin's moisture, or agitate yin's stillness. Paradoxically, yin and yang can also become each other, and rely on each other. Their relationship is not simply mutually consumptive." In terms of fertility, the inside of the uterus is yin; the moment the egg is released from the ovary would be yang.

According to nurse practitioner, fellowship graduate, and acupuncturist Ta-Ya Lee, "American women are typically on the go so much that often the yin, or quality of stillness, is neglected. When we struggle to have a baby, we keep trying, doing, and searching, but that is a yang approach. We need to slow down and honor our yin. To build up the yin, one needs to sleep well, or occasionally take a day off and simply do nothing. Forming a uterine nest is a yin creation."

TCM practitioners don't overrely on FSH lab results. A high FSH correlates with diminishing yin; if they can promote the yin, the FSH often comes down. Some women under the care of TCM practitioners conceive with what is considered an "infertile" FSH level of 25 to 30. Instead, practitioners keep an eye on the midcycle cervical fluid, which is an important indicator of fertility. Premature ovarian failure is also seen as a call to nourish yin.

The Three Vital Substances

In addition to the forces of yin and yang, TCM addresses and rectifies problems with the vital substances: qi, blood, and essence. Qi is not easily defined, and is often oversimplified as "energy." Perhaps it is better understood by its functions: to warm, to move, to transform, to contain, and to lift. The Chinese characters for qi include two symbols—one for rice, and the one for steam—signifying that qi is on the edge between material and immaterial metabolic processes, involving change at a cellular level. Qi is the driver of these metabolic processes. Blood is fluid and yin, nourishing the body and mind. Essence governs growth and reproduction, involves both yin and yang qualities, and declines with age.

The TCM practitioner assesses and treats problems with deficiency, stagnation, or lack of free and easy flow, primarily of qi or blood. The concept of depletion, which seems intuitive to most of us, is not yet part of Western medical thought; however, it is central to TCM. Depletion is more than fatigue. It is a state of chronic exhaustion, a lack of energy, and difficulty in mustering a response to life's challenges. Imagine for a moment the exact opposite of vitality, and you will understand depletion. If your body is depleted, it's harder to conceive because from an evolutionary perspective, the body realizes that you barely have the reserves to support your own organism, much less another, new one. So we not only need an abundance of these three substances but also need them to operate and move properly.

In Chinese medicine, we are born with a fixed amount of kidney qi or prenatal (i.e., inherited from our parents) qi. Dr. Jingduan Yang is a psychiatrist, fellowship graduate, and a fourth-generation teacher and international expert on classic forms of TCM. He typically assesses whether there is a deficiency of qi, and if there is, decides how to correct it. Kidney qi deficiency is the main factor in infertility; it can manifest as cold hands and feet, light periods, chronic back pain, and even early symptoms of menopause. A woman needs adequate kidney energy in order to conceive; too much anxiety or fear will also block the kidney qi.

The liver is responsible for making sure that things are moving, and liver qi stagnation is the second-most-common pattern that Dr. Yang sees in his practice. Typically a woman will present with symptoms of irritable bowel syndrome, fibromyalgia, migraine headaches, dysmenorrhea, or depression. If liver qi is stagnant, then the kidney energy will be secondarily blocked. The third most common pattern that he sees is spleen qi deficiency, which affects absorption, digestion, and metabolism. This woman may present with a slow metabolism, fatigue, muscle aches, trouble sleeping, and a tendency to worry. With spleen qi deficiency, one craves both sugar and sleep. In order to remedy this situation, dietary changes and exercise are vital. To make things even more complex, a person can have a combination of these various deficiencies, which only an expert TCM practitioner will be able to diagnose.

Movement of the Vital Substances

In order to be healthy and fertile, women need enough qi, blood, and essence, but also proper movement of these vital substances. Qi is responsible for transitioning the blood to create the menstrual cycle. Essence maintains ovaries and fertility, and a balance of yin and yang affects every aspect of health. Because reproduction depends upon kidney energy and essence, anything that a person can do to protect that energy is helpful. Lifestyle can greatly influence fertility. The amount and quality of kidney energy depends upon three factors:

1. how much kidney energy was inherited from one's parents (prenatal kidney energy)

2. lifestyle (Sexual behavior utilizes kidney energy; it consumes and depletes kidney energy. Therefore, when attempting to conceive, it is recommended to preserve the sexual energy for the purpose of increasing chances of pregnancy. This would translate to having sexual intercourse only around the time of ovulation. Dr. Yang explains how Chinese medicine proscribes the proper frequency of sexual activity, depending upon the age and the individual. For a thirty-year-old man, perhaps three times a week is fine; for some people, once a week may be too much. It depends on how much kidney energy a person has. In addition, Dr. Yang says that it's best not to have intercourse if one is

very tired, sick, or does not have enough time to relax beforehand. He also recommends having less sex in the winter, when kidney energy needs to be preserved and cultivated.)

3. emotional distress, especially fear, which affects kidney energy

TCM and the Menstrual Cycle

Traditional Chinese medicine describes elaborate theories of the physiology of the menstrual cycle. The menses are governed by the lunar month—gathering blood, getting ready for pregnancy, and then releasing. Leslie McGee says that "Women are human displays of cosmic forces." The menstrual cycle is considered the report card in Chinese medicine, and in the initial consultation, the practitioner asks detailed questions about it, as well as about the woman's lifestyle, medical history, diet, stress levels, and what she has tried in order to conceive.

The TCM practitioner pays particular attention to the color, quality, and quantity of menstrual blood, as these details provide telling clues. The color of the blood can indicate pathology; for instance, a purple flow indicates stasis, and often is accompanied by pain. Scant blood flow means that there is inadequate blood, which is an issue as women age. Or periods can become heavier as women get older. These abnormal patterns need to be corrected in order for fertility to be optimal. If the menstrual blood is sticky and dark, the uterine lining will not serve as a welcoming place for an embryo to implant. If a woman's period is very light, then yin is deficient; too heavy a flow means that there is a yang, or qi, deficiency. If the qi is weak, then blood can't be held in. All such problems must be corrected if the uterus is to house a growing fetus for nine months.

Stress

One of acupuncturist Leslie McGee's Chinese teachers said to her, "I can see that Americans are very stressed. In China, a family of four crowded into a two-room apartment is not as anxious as a family living in a large house here [in the United States]." It's true that in other countries, people often feel much less pressured than we do in America. Somehow we have allowed ourselves to become a nation of stressed-out individuals.

In Chinese medicine, stress is equated with excessive emotional distress and is considered a major impediment to conception. Too much fear, anger, sadness, loss, grief, worry, and resentment—or a combination of these—can affect different energetic systems in the body.

In TCM, each organ is associated with an emotion. Dr. Yang believes that in our society, women often don't get enough nurturing, on top of having quite a lot of responsibility. The liver doesn't handle stress well, and this presents as stagnation. To relieve stress, he recommends practicing mindful meditation and qi gong exercises (slow, graceful movements and controlled breathing techniques to promote circulation of qi).

As TCM practitioner Ta-Ya Lee says, "Many women today have type A personalities, and are under a lot of pressure. You have to practice letting go of some things. Look at how full your calendar is, and cut back on weekend activities. If you're a runner, slow down and walk. Qi gong exercises, breathing exercises, and meditation are helpful. Too much adrenaline makes it hard to conceive, and worry drains the spleen and kidney energy that is trying to hold the baby. Overwork is a huge factor in miscarriage."

Actively reducing stress so that the qi flows properly can be helpful in avoiding miscarriage. Leslie McGee recommends that women who conceive again after a prior miscarriage take two weeks off from work at the point at which they miscarried, to just relax until that particular stage of the pregnancy has passed.

TCM in Practice

Joe is a graduate of the Arizona Center for Integrative Medicine fellowship program. When he was doing his internal medicine internship, his brother and sister-in-law, who lived one block away, became pregnant. Then coincidentally, Joe and his wife, Heidi, conceived, but miscarried at twelve weeks.

"Even though the pregnancy was unplanned, when there was no heartbeat on the twelve-week ultrasound, it was devastating. And we had just started telling people that we were pregnant," Joe says.

Soon after the miscarriage, Heidi began to have dysmenorrhea and pain, and even passed out a few times; she was discovered to have endometriosis throughout her pelvis, but the gynecologist recommended trying to get pregnant before having surgery.

"It was devastating to lose our first baby, and bittersweet to watch my sister daily progressing, then delivering my healthy niece. Already I felt like a failure as a woman; then I am diagnosed with endometriosis. The fear that we might not be able to have a child of our own spurred me into action to find something to help us conceive."

Rather than surgery, Heidi decided to try acupuncture, since Western medicine didn't have a viable solution for her. She went to an acupuncturist who said, "I can work with you." She began treatment with acupuncture and Chinese herbs; within two months, Heidi's periods were pain-free and regular. Also notable was how other things stabilized. Heidi's hands and feet had always been extremely cold, but they became warm. The acupuncturist told her not to try to conceive until she'd had twelve months of treatments combined with herbs, in order to prepare her body for pregnancy. After a full year of needling and herbal remedies, Heidi got pregnant within one month of trying. She continued with the acupuncture throughout her pregnancy.

Joe and Heidi were very nervous through the first trimester, but the twelve-week ultrasound looked great. "When we saw the ultrasound, I felt elated, like all we had gone through and the work we had done to achieve this pregnancy had been for that moment," Heidi said. "Our son Gus brings us joy every day, and we are grateful for all of the things that made him possible." Joe credits his interest in integrative medicine with his positive experiences with TCM through Heidi's pregnancy.

Keeping the Pelvic Area Warm

Chinese medicine advises us to keep our feet warm, since the feet are equated with kidney energy, and the kidneys are close to the uterus. TCM practitioners recommend wearing socks and shoes, and avoiding walking barefoot on a tile floor. Ta-Ya

Lee also advises against going outside with wet hair to prevent cold invasion. It is thought that cold makes a person more vulnerable, so one should try to keep body temperature very even.

Most important, women are advised to keep the pelvic area warm. TCM describes two important energy centers in the body: the Ming Men, called the Gate of Life, is along the lower back, just above the hip bones. The Dan Tian (Center of Gravity or Red Field) is located between the navel and the pubic bone. A surprising number of women with fertility challenges have a cold abdominal area. These centers can be kept warm with a warm hot water bottle or heating pad (not electric) on the pelvic area or by warm clothes. Another strategy is to ask your partner to heat up the area with their hands in the same loving way we place our hands on the lower abdomen when a baby is gestating.

Practitioners might also warm the area through moxibustion, in which the herb *Artemesia vulgaris* is rolled into a cigar shape and lit. The flame is then put out, and the heat of the herb is brought to various acupressure points (without touching the body), in order to bring additional energy to those points.

Diet

Dietary considerations are important in Chinese medicine. Some of the ideas presented will sound quite foreign to Western ears, such as eating black foods to support kidney energy. Others seem to emerge from a time before refrigeration, when eating cooked food produced less health risk. Most, but not all, of the recommendations mesh well with those in the earlier chapter on nutrition.

Overall, TCM practitioners recommend eating a balanced omnivorous diet. If a woman is vegetarian, she is advised to eat eggs and dairy, and perhaps some chicken broth to support the essence, which benefits from animal proteins.

TCM places a high value on being able to digest foods well. Warm or cooked food is thought to be easier to digest and assimilate than raw food. Eating cooked food helps to provide the body with the qi it needs, whereas raw food moves the energy away from the kidneys, toward the digestive tract. Leslie McGee reminds us that when you eat ice-cold foods, your body has to warm the food up to 98.6 degrees in order to digest it. And while many women think that eating a lot of salads is healthy, TCM practitioners are wary of too many salads since they are composed of raw, cold ingredients.

Other foods to be avoided are those that are said to be "dampening." This includes whole wheat, white flour, and sugary or high-fructose foods; perhaps surprisingly, it also includes modern manufactured soy products. Tempeh, miso, and edamame are acceptable, but tofu should be eaten only in moderation.

Another issue is that people who eat the Standard American Diet have become extremely overheated and damp internally due to eating fried or high-fructose foods. Drinking freshly pressed juices from pure fruits and vegetables can help to correct that condition. Chinese medicine does not recommend fasting, perhaps because the Chinese people experienced famine as a society, but practitioners do advise avoiding overly rich foods. Whole-fat dairy, however, is thought to support fertility and the essence, while low-fat is associated with lack of ovulation.

Finally, in order to nourish kidney energy, practitioners recommend eating sea cucumbers, shrimp, and lamb, especially in winter when it is cold. Similarly, drinking fresh ginger tea is advised for its warming effect. Also good to consume are black beans, black sesame seeds, and black rice—indeed, any dark foods, since black is the color of the kidneys, and thus these foods support kidney energy.

Acupuncture

In Chinese medicine, the body is crisscrossed by a web of meridians, which are channels through which qi circulates. The acupuncture points are locations where the channels' qi rises to the skin's surface. There are twelve main meridians, six of which are yin; six, yang. The meridians form a network of energy channels throughout the body, and each is related to an organ or function.

An acupuncturist uses needles at points along the meridians to regulate the body's balance, and to enhance fertility. TCM theory holds that if a condition is long-standing or deep-seated, it will take awhile for acupuncture to work. In China, acupuncture would typically be done daily; while this is impractical in the United States, strive to have treatments twice a week. I usually recommend that women have six to eight visits before they assess the value of the treatments. With regard to fertility, a practitioner will need to observe a woman's pulses through a complete menstrual cycle to fully evaluate her. Preferably this is done before beginning any medication, as once a woman is on fertility medicine, it is difficult to tell what her original deficiency might be.

There are three postulated mechanisms for how acupuncture enhances fertility. The first is that it may mediate the release of neurotransmitters, leading the hypothalamus to release gonadotrophin-releasing hormone (GnRH), which stimulates the pituitary and then the ovaries. In this way, acupuncture might directly influence your menstrual cycle, ovulation, and overall fertility. Second, acupuncture may increase blood flow to the uterus by inhibiting activity in the uterine central sympathetic nervous system. Anything that brings more blood to the endometrium is believed to increase fertility. Third, acupuncture is believed to stimulate the production of endogenous opioids, which are the body's own pain inhibitors, and which could modify the body's stress response. Essentially, acupuncture works to create an overall relaxation response in the body.

Women who want to conceive can use acupuncture to improve their chances of success. As Leslie McGee says, "Ideally, someone will come to me earlier with the attitude of 'Help me be as fertile as possible,' as opposed to 'Tune me up within three weeks' time.' But in either case, I figure out a way to work with them. Some of my clients have done IVF and are exhausted from the process; in addition, their periods are messed up after the drugs. The IVF drugs are ovary stimulating, and are very hot; they push the ovaries to do the yang thing, which is to pop out an egg. Yet these hot medicines can damage the yin; the uterine lining can become too thin, and the cervical fluid dries up.

"In addition, a woman who uses Lupron, or other estrogen-blocking medication, can go into temporary menopause, so using the IVF drugs has its downside. Women who truly are cold often feel fine on these drugs; women with internal heat can feel awful. Using Chinese medicine to enhance fertility when taking a break from IVFs can have a very positive effect."

We are learning more all the time about acupuncture combined with IVF. A meta-analysis, or review that combined the information from several studies (in this case, seven), was done with 1,356 women who used acupuncture to complement an IVF procedure. The meta-analysis included only studies where acupuncture was performed on either the day before or after the embryo transfer. Most commonly, acupuncture was done twenty-five minutes before the transfer, and then immediately after. The study showed a significant increase in clinical pregnancy, ongoing pregnancy, and live birth. There was a 65 percent increase in the likelihood of becoming pregnant if acupuncture was used along with an embryo transfer. More important, there was a 91 percent increase in live births. I would strongly advocate that you look for a clinic that offers acupuncture, as it is inexpensive compared to IVF, enhances the odds of conceiving, reduces stress, and improves overall well-being.

Dr. Paul Magarelli is a reproductive endocrinologist in Colorado Springs whose wife is an acupuncturist. The protocol at their clinic is to do acupuncture for four weeks before egg retrieval, two sessions per week. Then on the day of the transfer, they follow the protocol of Dr. Wolfgang Paulus, who performed the pioneering research that showed improved conception rates in women undergoing IVF who had acupuncture twenty-five minutes prior to and immediately after the time of embryo transfer.

Dr. Magarelli did a retrospective analysis of 576 IVF cycles in his practice. Acupuncture beginning four weeks prior to IVF resulted in 26 percent more pregnancies than did IVF with acupuncture pre- and post-transfer alone. Magarelli also measured serum cortisol and serum prolactin in the run-up to the retrieval, and found significant changes in the acupuncture group. Going through IVF increases anxiety, which affects the hypothalamic pituitary axis and causes hormonal changes; acupuncture can reduce these negative effects of stress.

In a small study, twenty infertile Australian women were asked about their experiences after four or more acupuncture sessions. Acupuncture was perceived to have a positive impact on health. The results also suggested that further studies should look at resiliency, anxiety, and well-being, all of which seemed to be positively affected by the acupuncture treatments. Indeed, many of my patients describe a deep sense of relaxation as a result of acupuncture sessions. They describe it as a "time-out," "a healing time," and their "time for self-care and for balancing."

Julie is someone who hated needles but was determined to do everything it took to become pregnant. When she was in her midthirties, after being told that there was a 15 to 20 percent chance of IVF working, and a 2 percent chance of conceiving on her own, she decided to proceed with IVF. For her first two transfers, she worked with a fertility clinic and no TCM practitioners. The first produced only three embryos, and the second, two; Julie did not conceive with either procedure, as none of the embryos were of good quality. At the time, she was seeing a craniosacral practitioner, who "practically insisted" that she see Dr. Jingduan Yang. Despite her strong aversion to needles, Julie agreed to give TCM a try.

Dr. Yang diagnosed low kidney energy and recommended acupuncture and Chinese herbs. Julie had acupuncture two or three times a week for four weeks leading up to the third IVF transfer. She also took herbs prescribed by Dr. Yang in pill and tea forms. This time Julie produced two good embryos and did conceive. She continued with the acupuncture for the first twelve weeks of pregnancy. Her precious child is now two years old.

Julie eventually tried two more IVFs, but the new fertility clinic did not allow the herbs, and she feels that this might have been a factor in her not conceiving then. However, she was thrilled to become pregnant with a donor egg, having used acupuncture during that procedure. As Julie says, "No matter how you get there, it's all good. Having a child is a true gift."

Laura (a pseudonym) used a combination of yoga, acupuncture, and meditation to enhance her fertility. She reports,

> I got into yoga and meditation initially in 2002; I had a stressful job as a criminal prosecutor, and did it to deal with my stress and also the back pain from an injury when I was a teenager. I had a good yoga teacher who started me on a path of meditation; she also later referred me to an acupuncturist. In addition, my first husband and I were trying to get pregnant, and we did an unsuccessful IVF when I was thirty-two. The fertility doctors focused more on my husband's issues, and ignored the fact that I was having a very short luteal phase. Our marriage was under great strain from the infertility, and eventually it ended.
>
> When I was thirty-four, I started acupuncture for the back pain and stress, even though I was very afraid of needles. However, the

needles didn't hurt, and I felt that the treatment really released the pain, and also helped me on an emotional and spiritual level. I had switched to civil prosecution, which was less stressful than criminal, but I was working fifty-hour weeks. (The criminal job was eighty hours a week.) I also maintained a regular yoga and meditation practice. This I engaged in primarily for stress reduction and spiritual growth, and because I find it a very healthy practice and outlook for people in my profession.

As I got older, my cycles shortened to twenty-one to twenty-three days, and I became concerned that I wouldn't be able to have children. I began seeing Dr. Lee, a Chinese acupuncturist in San Francisco. She was the first person to tell me that I was too hot, and that my body's heat was shortening my cycle. She gave me herbs twice a day to cool me down, and also put a needle below my navel and heated the top of it. The acupuncture and herbs helped lengthen my cycle; she dealt with an issue that no one else had addressed in seven years. Dr. Lee also felt that I had too many toxins in my body from the ibuprofen I took for back pain, and the diet sodas I drank, so I stopped consuming those things.

I met my second husband, and for a year we tried to conceive, with no luck. Then we moved and I went back to my first acupuncturist, who had begun to focus on fertility. In addition to regular treatments, she referred me to a naturopath, and this was a big break for me. The naturopath helped me to totally detoxify; she prescribed a series of homeopathic remedies as well as chlorella (algae), ground flaxseed, and licorice to cleanse and build up my blood. My cycle lengthened to twenty-eight days, and I began to ovulate earlier. She was also the first practitioner to tell me to stop taking antihistamines for allergies, because they were drying up my cervical mucus.

Within six months of combining the naturopath's treatments with acupuncture, at age thirty-nine, I got pregnant, and my son was born seven weeks ago. I call him the "ten-year baby" because of everything I went through waiting to conceive. But he was worth the wait!

Miscarriage

Chinese medicine also has suggestions for women who miscarry easily. Miscarriage is often related to weak kidney and spleen energy, and the emotional reaction after a miscarriage affects the kidney, liver, and spleen qi. Since one of the functions of qi is holding, TCM practitioners use herbs and acupuncture to protect and contain the baby.

One of Leslie McGee's clients—we'll call her Joanne—had had two devastating miscarriages; she would conceive, but couldn't stay pregnant. Joanne felt that, rather than spend the money on IVF, she would start the adoption process. Two weeks after being chosen by a young pregnant woman who was making an adoption plan, Joanne herself unexpectedly became pregnant.

Leslie worked with Joanne to sustain the pregnancy and to bolster her spirits; following her miscarriages, Joanne found it hard to fully trust in her pregnancy. She did go on to adopt a baby, and then when this infant was five months old, her biological baby was born. It's an amazing story; Joanne now has two children, born five months apart. Her experience is a wonderful reminder that if the goal is becoming a mother, there are many paths to getting there.

Herbs

When there is not enough qi, blood, or essence, often a TCM practitioner will prescribe herbs. These herbal combinations, given in either capsule form or tea, were generated long ago by Chinese doctors; today, a TCM practitioner might modify them a bit, but will basically follow the time-tested formulae.

Never choose Chinese herbs for yourself—knowing how to use various herbs synergistically is a lifelong learning process. A trained TCM doctor should prescribe them after evaluating your condition and checking to see what other medications you are taking, to avoid interactions with any Western medicines.

A typical herbal mixture might include ten or twelve herbs to build the blood and improve fertility. Days 1–14 (approximately) are the follicular phase of a woman's cycle; during follicle growth, practitioners use herbs that keep body temperature low and nourish the yin. Days 15–28 are the luteal phase when progesterone should dominate, so warming herbs are added.

Herbs transform different energy channels and affect energy in a similar way to acupuncture. The herbs prescribed will depend on the practitioner's assessment of the major deficiency or stagnation. Herbs may be an excellent strategy for women who want to use natural methods to enhance fertility before trying to conceive. Small studies show the benefits of Chinese herbs for endometriosis, PCOS, and dysmenorrhea. Trained clinicians report great success across a wide range of women's health issues.

However, many reproductive endocrinologists and ob-gyns are uncomfortable with using herbs along with their hormonal treatments. They worry about interactions that might interfere with reported success rates. This concern is justifiable from the perspective that many of the Chinese herbal formulas have not yet been studied. Some women (and doctors) will be comfortable with this uncertainty; others will not.

One encouraging study of Chinese herbs added them to the ovulation-inducing medication Clomid. The women who received the herbal formulas along with Clomid had thicker uterine lining, better-quality cervical mucus, and a conception rate of 41 percent. This was a significant improvement over the women in the control group, who were given only Clomid and had a conception rate of 22 percent.

Men

While fewer men seek out Chinese medicine for fertility issues, practitioners often find the same deficiencies in kidney energy so common in women. Western medicine typically assesses only sperm count, quality, and mobility. But even if a man's sperm count is normal, TCM theorizes that he needs good kidney energy in order to conceive, and therefore uses herbs and acupuncture to balance the kidney qi.

Using TCM to Enhance Fertility

It will probably come as no surprise that I am a strong advocate of including traditional Chinese medicine in our approach when couples are struggling with their fertility. TCM is not something you will practice on yourself; you will need to visit a skilled practitioner to see if you are a good candidate for acupuncture or for herbal remedies.

Still, many of its principles can be applied. Ask yourself, what can I do to bring my body into greater harmony? What might you remove from your to-do list to have better balance and more yin time? Can you enhance your kidney qi (and thus your reproductive capacity) by managing emotional stress and anger, and by clearing up lingering relationship challenges? What about eating more warm and cooked foods, and fewer raw or cold choices? Might you begin a ritual in which you warm your Ming-Men and Dan-Tian centers daily? Following these self-care practices are simple ways to bring the spirit and wisdom of Chinese medicine into your quest for a healthy child.

CHAPTER 9

AYURVEDA

Ayurveda, Sanskrit for "the science of life," is a system of traditional medicine native to India. One woman I know, Falguni Shah, described to me how Ayurveda played a part in her fertility journey.

Falguni was raised in a home that practiced the Hindu faith and followed Ayurvedic practices. This commitment to her tradition led Falguni to embrace an Ayurvedic approach when she and her husband decided to have a baby. She had a strong belief in a natural way of living, and in the principle of cleansing and preparing the body, mind, and spirit before bringing a child into the world.

A year before trying to conceive, Falguni and her husband met with their family priest, who performed a Hindu ceremony setting out the intention to bring a new soul to life. They prayed that "If there is meant to be a new soul, let us please be the vessel for it." Three months before starting to try to get pregnant, they began practicing abstinence so their energy and intention would be stronger and purer. Soon after, they realized they were not quite ready to get pregnant yet, and the couple wound up being abstinent for almost a year. In hindsight, Falguni felt that this year of abstinence strengthened their relationship.

The couple also consulted with a Hindu astrologer who read their charts in order to figure out the best time for them to conceive. He gave Falguni and her husband a mantra to recite daily. They recited it for twenty minutes each morning for five months and meditated together as well. Falguni says that this "mental preparation for having a child also pushed her to work with her husband to make their relationship stronger, and their communication better."

Dr. Vasant Lad of the Ayurvedic Institute in Albuquerque, New Mexico, had taught Falguni how to do home *panchakarma,* a form of detoxification. During this cleansing process, she ate a mono diet that included only lentils and rice; practiced external oleation by massaging herself with oils; and used herbal-infused oil enemas to rid her body of toxins. Both members of the couple took herbs to aid fertility: Falguni's herb was *shatavari*; her husband's, *ashwaganda,* or Indian ginseng. They conceived their daughter with ease, and she was born through natural childbirth.

While Falguni's preparation for pregnancy may seem extreme to most, it serves to demonstrate the richness of traditional societies' approaches to preparing for new life. Ayurveda may be even more complex than traditional Chinese medicine, and is far less familiar to those of us in the West. It is not yet licensed as a modality in the United States, and there are fewer practitioners. While most of us have heard of concepts such as yin and yang, and qi, fewer of us know the three body constitutions, or doshas, central to Ayurvedic theories. More familiar, and closely linked to the practice of Ayurveda, is yoga, which can play a central role in fertility.

Western medicine is often referred to as "traditional," but Ayurveda, which is five thousand years old, is traditional in the truest sense of the word, as is Chinese medicine. At about 150 years old, Western medicine is actually the newcomer on the scene. Dating back to 3000 BC, Ayurveda exists not only as an oral tradition but also as a comprehensive written medical system recorded in Sanskrit texts. Ayurveda encompasses a complex view of human life as an inseparable union of body, mind, and spirit.

In Ayurveda, the body's constitutional health, or *prakruti,* involves a balanced state of the three energies, or doshas; the seven bodily tissues; proper digestion and disposal of waste matter; and a joyful and satisfied state of the senses, mind, and spirit. Body and mind must find a sense of contentment, because discontent is considered the root of disease and illness. Each person has a unique place of balance; the goal is to reach and maintain this centered state.

I have visited India twice, the second time as part of a delegation of U.S. integrative medicine educators and researchers. Invited by the National Institute of Ayurveda, Yoga, Unani, Siddha, and Homeopathy (AYUSH), I had an opportunity to visit one of the 450 Ayurvedic medical colleges and the National Institute of Yoga as well as many Ayurvedic hospitals and clinics. India has Western doctors and institutions as well as Ayurvedic, homeopathic, and other traditional systems including Siddha and Unani. The population is discriminating, choosing Western medicine for acute infections or surgical conditions, but often selecting traditional healing systems to treat chronic illness that results from an unhealthy lifestyle. For example, a woman might see an Ayurvedic physician for PCOS; for a blocked tube, she would visit a Western doctor.

Vata, Pitta, and Kapha

The three doshas, or fundamental principles within human beings, are Vata, Pitta, and Kapha. As I describe them, notice whether any seem to resonate; they may describe you or someone you know well. The first dosha, Vata, is associated with space and air, and with the principle of movement. Anything that has to do with motion, or lack thereof, is related to Vata.

Vata is necessary for thinking, breathing, circulation, ingestion, elimination of wastes, menstruation, and childbirth. In addition, this dosha includes the qualities of dry, light, cold, rough, subtle, mobile, and clear. A Vata personality is a rapid thinker and talker, creative and enthusiastic, and a light sleeper. A person in whom this dosha is dominant would probably be very thin, with her mind in the clouds so often that she even forgets to eat. She needs to be more grounded in general, and to have set sleeping, waking, and eating times.

The second dosha, Pitta, is associated with fire and water—everything that can be

181

heated—and governs the principle of transformation. Pitta is responsible for metabolism, digestion, maintaining our body temperature, appetite, and thirst. Pitta also involves our intake of sound, as well as of ideas, and includes sharp, hot, light, liquid, mobile, oily, and penetrating qualities. A person in whom Pitta is the dominant dosha would have a medium frame and height, and would be a moderate sleeper and a quick and incisive thinker. Pitta types are creative, ambitious, and self-confident. Many leaders hold this quality.

Kapha is associated with earth, water, and stability. This dosha contributes to growth and nourishment, including bone and muscle structure; repair and regeneration; lubrication; stamina; sleep; and memory. The qualities of Kapha include heavy, cold, dull, oily, liquid, smooth, dense, soft, static, cloudy, hard, and usually moist as well. Kapha personalities are peacemakers; they are tolerant and patient and eager to lend a hand. Their very "groundedness" makes them sound sleepers who tend to have large builds and slow-moving bodies.

While all three doshas exist to some extent in everyone, the amount varies widely from person to person. I, for instance, am Pitta dominant and have equal amounts of Kapha and Vata. You can determine your own dosha by answering a series of questions on the following Web site: www.banyanbotanicals.com/constitutions.

The Three Doshas

Vata

Necessary for: thinking, breathing, circulation, ingestion, elimination of wastes, menstruation, and childbirth

Qualities: dry, light, cold, rough, subtle, mobile, clear

Personality: rapid thinker and talker; creative and enthusiastic; light sleeper

Body type: thin

Pitta

Necessary for: metabolism, digestion, maintaining body temperature, appetite, and thirst

Qualities: fire, water; anything that can be heated; transformation

Personality: creative, ambitious, self-confident; a leader

Body type: medium frame and height

Kapha

Necessary for: growth and nourishment; repair and regeneration; lubrication, stamina, sleep, and memory

Qualities: earth, water, and stability

Personality: tolerant, patient, peacemaker, eager to help

Body type: heavy-set physique; strong bones and muscles

Prakruti: The Balance of the Doshas

Ayurvedic practitioners use a treatment approach of opposites to balance whatever is in excess or depleted. The goal is to reach one's own unique balanced constitutional state, or prakruti. A person's prakruti is determined at birth and remains constant throughout life. Prakruti can be dominant in one, two, or all three doshas, and no dosha is considered better or worse than another. Lifestyle choices regarding diet, exercise, good digestion, and processing of emotions can help to preserve doshic balance, contributing to a greater sense of happiness.

In Ayurveda, *agni* means digestive fire, and it is the root of all health. Agni refers to gastrointestinal digestion and also includes what is absorbed through the skin, the respiratory system, and even emotional experiences. Thus agni processes not only food but also all experiences, including those involving family and work. If what is ingested is good, agni can transform it into nourishment for the body, mind, and spirit. If unhealthy things are taken in, this results in *ama,* or toxic buildup.

When we are in balance, we get nourishment from healthy things, with unhealthy matter being removed in our wastes. Regular bowel movements are very important to make sure that *prana* (or the flow of energy) is functioning at optimal levels. If ama becomes too extensive, then Ayurveda calls for more moderation in our diet, stressors, lifestyle, and toxins, so that our bodies can return to an optimal state. If there isn't proper flow, stagnation results, which can lead to imbalance and disease.

Strikingly, Ayurveda has specific lifestyle recommendations for every part of the day; these vary, depending on your predominant doshas. In general, we are advised to follow the forty-two steps of *dinacharya,* which is loosely defined as the wisdom of one's day or ideal routine. For instance, in the morning it is recommended that you awaken before sunrise, because the hours between three and seven a.m. are the best time to receive divine knowledge, to study, and to meditate. It is held that you are more receptive to visions, revelations, and dream therapy at this time of day.

Before meditating, you are advised to attend to the purity of your body: using the bathroom, taking dosha-specific herbs, and cleaning your mouth, eyes, throat, lungs, and nose (using a Neti pot). Brushing your teeth before eating prevents you from ingesting germs from the previous night. In addition, scraping your tongue with a copper tongue scraper reduces phlegm. Drinking a mug of warm water clears out mucus in the throat. Next, you might chant to clear your body's channels, and then do gentle exercise such as walking or gardening, followed by *abhyanga* (self-massage) with oils. Oils are always used instead of lotions, since your body would ingest the paraffins and other chemicals in lotions.

Following abhyanga, you would eat a small amount of food, and then meditate for about fifteen minutes, using the style of meditation and mantra that was assigned for your dosha. Next you'd eat breakfast, dress in clothing made of natural fabrics, and declutter your home to rid it of ama (toxins).

Ayurveda also prescribes a comprehensive set of moral practices and good conduct, instructions for how to behave in the world, and for how the mind should think. These ethical guidelines, *yamas* and *niyamas,* are part of the eight limbs of yoga. They are recommended to put one's mind in a good framework.

The yamas, or social behaviors, include avoiding excess; not stealing or being possessive; and being truthful and nonviolent. The niyamas, or observances and restraints, encompass self-study and self-discipline, surrender, purity, and contentment.

Ayurveda and Fertility

To address fertility issues, an Ayurvedic practitioner assesses a person's system as a whole, including the condition of the three doshas, as well as agni and ama. If any of the doshas are imbalanced, reproductive problems may ensue. For instance, if one cannot digest well (a Pitta imbalance), then agni and ama are affected, which could result in infertility. According to Tanmeet Sethi, MD, a family physician, fellowship graduate, and faculty member at the Swedish Cherry Hill Family Medicine Residency, "Everything you eat, do, and ingest impacts fertility. Meditation, stress reduction, and digestive fire are all very important."

Dr. Sethi, who studied Ayurveda at the Ayurvedic Academy in Seattle and through an apprenticeship in India, begins an assessment by figuring out what imbalance is causing or exacerbating the infertility. She considers whether it relates to dietary issues, poor nutrition, emotional issues, or imbalance in sexual activity, among other concerns. She seeks to discover the nature of a woman's relationship with her partner—whether it is loving and nurturing, and if there was any trauma earlier in life that could be causing blockages. If so, counseling and mind-body medicine tools are recommended. According to Premal Patel, MD, a family physician who trained at the Ayurveda Institute in Albuquerque, proper bodily flow is a critical part of reproductive health for both men and women. Fertility depends on the *shukra* (male tissues) or *arthava* (female tissues) receiving proper nutrition. Nutrition moves through seven layers of tissues, or *dhatus*: through the circulatory system, then the adipose and nervous systems. Ultimately nourishment arrives at the deepest, which is the reproductive system. The other tissues must be healthy and unblocked, and the blood must be optimally cleansed, in order for nutrients to pass through all seven dhatus successfully.

185

The Menstrual Cycle

As in TCM, the quality of the menstrual cycle is a window into a woman's overall health. The practitioner will question if the menses occur at appropriate intervals; are not too dark or too bright; have no foul odor or clots; and lack mucus, pain, or cramping.

Each part of the menstrual cycle is generated by a different dosha. Kapha produces the follicular phase; Pitta, the luteal; and Vata is the descending wind that empties the uterus through menstruation. Any disturbance of dosha could affect fertility, but most commonly Vata is the problem. A Vata imbalance might present with scanty menses and irregular or skipped cycles, as well as old or brownish blood, cramping, and pain. Pitta issues would present as more profuse bleeding, sharpness, burning, and short intervals of menstruation. Kapha involvement would cause profuse bleeding; mucusy, liquid menses; as well as PMS symptoms, such as a sense of heaviness, grouchiness, and depression.

Ayurvedic medicine considers PCOS a disorder involving all three doshas. Weight reduction would be advised, as it is in Western medicine. Herbs might also be recommended, such as fenugreek to reduce blood sugar, and ashwaganda to reduce stress. One study found that Ayurveda could be helpful in PCOS through controlling diet, weight reduction, and herb supplementation.

Diet

Diet is central to Ayurvedic practice. Overall, we are advised to eat only until the stomach is half-full of food, leaving one quarter of the stomach to be filled with liquid and one quarter with air. Whenever possible, we are to consume fresh, organic foods and to avoid canned or frozen foods. There are complex seasonal recommendations involving types and temperature of foods, levels of spiciness, and cleansing and fasting with vegetable juices. In general, half of total food consumption should be fresh fruits and vegetables (an ancient recommendation that perfectly matches the new USDA choosemyplate.gov dietary recommendations). Whole grains such as wheat, barley, and rice are also beneficial, as is mung dal (split lentils) for protein.

Hot, spicy foods; sour or acidic dishes; heavily fermented foods; and peppers, onions, and garlic are all to be avoided because these can hinder fertility and lead to miscarriage. If you are a meat eater, choose antibiotic- and hormone-free meats, and avoid cold cuts and fast food.

Some foods that Ayurvedic practitioners consider particularly favorable for enhancing fertility include almonds or walnuts that have been soaked in water overnight; fresh juicy fruits such as mangoes, pears, plums, and peaches; and dried fruits including dates, figs, and raisins. In addition, bananas cooked with cardamom and ghee and high-quality lentils and grains are good for promoting conception.

To balance Vata, Ayurvedic practitioners advise avoiding cold or raw foods, and switching to nourishing, warming, cooked foods. For Pitta balance, use soothing, cooling foods, adding spices such as fennel and aloe vera. With Kapha imbalance, consume warm foods that are lighter in nature, and avoid cheeses, yogurt, milk, and other mucus-producing foods.

Herbal Remedies

Often an Ayurvedic practitioner will recommend herbs to regulate the menstrual cycle before a woman tries to conceive. While cooking herbs—cumin, turmeric, and fennel—are alright to use without seeing a practitioner, it is best to use other herbs in consultation. Some herbs are used to help regulate the menstrual cycle, and are then stopped when a woman begins to attempt to conceive.

Throughout Indian history, shatavari (*Asparagus racemosus*) has been the principal herb for fertility. As discussed in "Supplements," *shatavari* means "she who possesses one hundred husbands" in Sanskrit, implying its ability to promote fertility and vitality. Shatavari tubers were once candied and eaten as a sweet; nursing mothers ate shatavari to support production of breast milk; and it was used in medicinal oils for its soothing and cooling properties. Shatavari is said to increase the attractive quality and robustness of the genital organs, to balance the pH in the cervix, and to be a general panacea for women's health.

The principal constituents of shatavari include saponins, alkaloids, proteins, and tannins. The plant contains triterpene saponins or shatavarin I-IV, which aid the body's natural production of estrogen. It supports healthy blood flow through the reproductive system as well as normal hormone utilization and blood hormone levels. Researchers at the Interdisciplinary School of Health Sciences, University of Pune in

India, also found that shatavari helps normalize white-blood-count levels and benefits immune and digestive system function.

Ashoka (*Saraca asoca*) is derived from the bark of the Ashoka tree, one of the sacred trees of India. Its medicinal importance has been described in various Ayurvedic scriptures. According to traditional stories, Sita, wife of Lord Rama, was kidnapped by the evil Ravana, and the Ashoka tree gave Sita comfort, strength, and support in her time of difficulty. *Ashoka* translates into "sorrowless" or "without grief"; it is therefore said to be a woman's friend. A woman's menses are also poetically described as the "weeping of the womb," so Ashoka helps with that "weeping" (menses). Fertility rituals were performed in which women painted their feet red and kicked the tree, passing on fecundity to its buds to make it flower. Today, the bark of the tree is used to cure excessive loss of blood during menstruation due to uterine fibroids and other problems.

Another herb commonly used by Ayurvedic practitioners is ashwaganda (*Withania somnifera*). Ashwaganda is sometimes called Indian ginseng because of its adaptogenic properties, which help the body adapt to stress. It aids in addressing Pitta issues in both men and women. In a three-month controlled study, a group of infertile men with normal sperm count who took the herb were compared to a control group of fertile men with normal sperm count. Taking 5 grams per day of ashwaganda caused a reduction in stress, raised levels of antioxidants, improved sperm quality, and resulted in a 14 percent pregnancy rate in the infertile men's partners. Additionally, cortisol levels dropped in the treated men, reducing the toll on the adrenal glands.

Another herb used for male infertility is *Mucuna pruriens,* which acts upon the hypothalamic pituitary gonadal axis. A study was done with seventy-five men who were being screened for infertility and seventy-five fertile men. Researchers measured serum thyroid, lutenizing hormone (LH), follicle stimulating hormone (FSH), prolactin, dopamine, adrenaline, and noradrenaline in seminal fluid and blood. After taking *Mucuna pruriens,* the men showed improved thyroid, LH, dopamine, adrenaline, and noradrenaline levels, as well as reduced FSH and prolactin levels. In addition, sperm count and motility were significantly improved after treatment.

Many other herbs are traditionally prescribed by Ayurvedic practitioners. Dr. Sethi uses cumin to purify the uterus; *ajwain,* or carom seeds, for stomach pain; and turmeric for its effects upon the interactions of hormones and tissues. Bhaswati Bhattacharya, MPH, MD, director of the Dinacharya Institute in New York City, which provides training in Ayurveda, dispenses *Trachelospermum,* cumin, turmeric, and black cumin to purify the genital tract. Fenugreek is used as an aphrodisiac and also to normalize blood sugar levels. Dr. Patel favors the herb Triphala Guggulu for Kapha involvement, but it must be discontinued once the person is attempting to conceive. For men, all three doctors use *guduchi,* another adaptogen, to enhance overall genital health.

The Role of Meditation, Prayer, and Yoga

Ayurveda promotes a satisfied and content state of mind, and considers a healthy body, mind, and spirit to be supremely important for optimal fertility. Meditation, yoga, breathing exercises, prayer, and journaling are recommended; the specific practice depends in part on one's dosha, but also on what appeals most to the individual patient, in order to reach a state of joyful contentment.

I was first introduced to yoga while living in San Francisco in the 1980s as a medical student and have had a regular practice ever since. I prefer a style called Anusara, which means "flowing with grace." Based in part on Iyengar yoga and in part on Vinyasa flow, it pays attention to alignment as well as to heart-centering practices. I have seen great benefit in my own life from this practice; my posture is straighter, and I feel much more centered. I often recommend yoga as a body-mind practice to my patients.

Linda Sparrowe is an internationally known yoga teacher and health expert, and the author of *The Woman's Book of Yoga and Health: A Lifelong Guide to Wellness.* She works with teacher-training programs, teaching new yoga instructors how to approach women who want to have healthy babies or who are dealing with infertility issues. I have had the privilege of teaching workshops together with Linda at the Shambhala Mountain Center in Colorado, and I love her instructional style.

Linda points out that "doctors can be pretty dismissive of women, saying, 'If you just relax, you will get pregnant.' Telling a stressed person to relax is like telling an angry, raging person to calm down—easy to say, and not so easy to do. By the time a woman confides her nervousness about pregnancy to her doctor, she's probably

189

already feeling anxious and maybe even disappointed and frustrated with her body. But yoga puts her into a relationship with her body that is nurturing and loving. For some women, practicing asana and breathing techniques is the only opportunity they have to see their body as an ally.

"The practice of yoga helps us get to know ourselves; to be comfortable with our bodies and what they are capable of; and to prepare our wombs. Yoga also puts us in touch with our emotions, allaying our fears or anxiety, and on a deeper energetic level, through conscious breathing exercises, helps us open our hearts and minds to the possibility of creating life. The more we practice asanas (poses) and pranayama (breathing exercises) with mindful intention, the more success we'll have."

According to Linda, the best yoga poses to enhance fertility include Upavishta Konasana, or seated forward fold pose, which causes the uterus to pull inward a bit. She instructs women to visualize lightly lifting the area between the perineum and the anus, without gripping or grabbing (much lighter than kegels). She feels that the Ardha Chandrasana is the quintessential pose for all women, especially those who want to get pregnant. Ardha Chandrasana (half-moon pose) is a balance pose. (With your weight on one leg and both hands on the ground, lift your other leg, keeping it straight, with your foot flexed, to hip height, and turn it to open the pelvis. If you feel stable, you can lift your arm, extending it to the sky.) This pose, which can also be done against the wall, helps you bring loving attention to your belly, without gripping, and allows you to breathe slowly and deeply into the womb.

Linda offers these ten pointers about the ways that yoga enhances fertility:

1. Yoga is a powerful stress reliever: When highly stressed, the body moves energy away from the reproductive system, making conception even more difficult. Yoga reduces stress, bringing the body and mind into alignment.

2. Befriending your body: Women who struggle with infertility or who have just had miscarriages are sad and disappointed, and often they are also angry with their bodies for betraying them. Yoga helps women get in touch with their bodies, not adversarially, but with compassion and understanding.

3. Proper Posture/Alignment: Pelvic floor misalignment can impede pregnancy. So can tight hips or a scooped tailbone. Any type of yoga that focuses on alignment can help promote *apana vayu*—the downward motion of energy that massages and prepares our uteruses for pregnancy. Yoga hip openers, twists, and inversions are helpful.

4. Open Heart/Open Womb: Gentle backbends (like Setu Bandhasana, while supported) can help calm, and bring healing energy to the belly. Yoga can help you to be open to possibilities and to notice when you start to close down around your fears.

5. Nurturing the pelvis: Seated poses such as Baddha Konasana and Upavistha Konasana are excellent ways of softening the belly, calming agitation, increasing circulation in the pelvic area, regulating menstrual flow, and stimulating the ovaries. Begin upright and then relax into a forward bend, resting your head on a block or bolster.

6. Cooling the brain: Any time you rest your head on something, you will calm the mind, and help balance the nervous system. You can do this in Adho Mukha Svanasana (downward-facing dog pose) and in forward bends.

7. Chanting the sound of "Om": Patanjali, author of the *Yoga Sutra*, wrote that chanting the syllable "Om" removes all obstacles to practice, helps turn your mind inward, and brings you right to the source of wisdom. You can chant "Om" or choose your own simple mantras: pick one (or even a couple of different ones) that will get you through difficult times, and another that can be a guiding light in your life. Let the mantra ride on the waves of the breath; let it be the vehicle to calm and nourish.

8. Deep breathing/pranayama practice: After miscarriage or when a woman is struggling to get pregnant, she doesn't always breathe into her belly—sometimes she avoids that part of her own body—breathing out of fear, anger, guilt, remorse. Soothing breaths bring life and nourishment to the womb—and help release anxiety and fear.

9. Pause when necessary: If you feel agitated or anxious during practice, pause or stop altogether and concentrate on your breath, with focused attention on the exhale to ground your energy. Bending forward, resting your head on a bolster or chair will calm your nerves as well.

10. Watch your language: How do you describe (out loud and to yourself) what you're going through? Do you think, I'm never going to have a baby, or can you say, I'm doing all I can to get pregnant? Do you "hate" your hips, chastise your belly, berate your uterus, or can you offer kindness, compassion, and healing breaths to those parts of you that need help? Remember that from space comes quiet; within the silence, look to your heart to find peace.

Please see "Additional Resources" for Linda's suggestions for the best poses to enhance fertility. Also worth noting are a few of her warnings: Linda advises against a rigorous yoga practice, as too intense a workout can be detrimental to reproductive health. She suggests that women treat themselves gently, doing sequences that feel luscious, connecting, and grounding. She also advises that women move away from more demanding aerobic practices, like Ashtanga or power yoga, toward a more mindful approach to asana. Finally, she warns against doing deep twists if you think there's a chance you could be pregnant. Twists signal the body to squeeze and expel—not the energetics you want to encourage if you are pregnant.

De West is a yoga teacher based in Boulder, Colorado, who works with many women throughout their fertility journeys. She highly recommends that you tell your teacher if you are trying to conceive, and the phase you are in, so that the asanas may be organized to support your needs. She says, "I like to break down the yoga practice with intention, emphasizing the mind-body connection. I tell the women in my classes to think about the messages they are sending to their bodies. It's not only about wanting a baby; it's also about cleaning up the garden and getting ready to plant; having a seed and holding it preciously."

In the follicular phase of a woman's cycle, she suggests a lot of inversions such as headstand (Sirsasana) and shoulder stand (Sarvangasana). These more advanced asanas are for a student who's been practicing for a while; more basic inversions can be done with support, using a chair, the wall, or wall ropes. Other asanas she recommends include standing poses that work on the rotation of the legs and femur bones and open the pelvis in all directions, thereby gently circulating blood flow to the pelvis. Pelvis openers in the seated position, she points out, can be done throughout a woman's whole life. De recommends half-moon pose (Ardha Chandrasana), which opens up the belly area, as well as triangle pose (Trikonasana), and side angle pose (Parsvakonasana).

"In the luteal phase, it is okay to do forward bends with an open belly; supported inversions that balance the reproductive and hormonal areas of body; restorative stress-reducing postures; and hip and pelvic openers to increase blood flow to the pelvis. Rather than gripping their abdomen, women need to create a flow of breath into the belly and pelvis. Forward bends are fine, especially downward dog with your head supported, resting head in your hands.

"There are certain poses that I tell women to avoid during the luteal phase," De says. "I don't want them to do any poses that compress or wring, and none that lift, squeeze, or loosen. You want to protect the egg and its support. Big backbends such as Dhanurasana, or bow pose, are not good because they are thinning and more active, energizing, and cleansing. Navasana (boat pose) is not good because it grips the abdomen.

"Once a woman is pregnant, if she has had an earlier miscarriage, I follow a certain protocol. In general, avoid standing poses and squatting poses because you don't want to send that message of evacuation to your body. Instead, I turn the body upside down to create a feeling of 'stay in there.' Forward bends, inversions, and seated poses are great; Baddha Konasana is fine as long as the thighs are supported. Restorative postures are key.

"Recently I worked with a triathlete in her early thirties who had one failed IVF, then tried to conceive for a year. We talked about things in her practice that might need to change. For instance, rather than a hot yoga class, I suggested a more cooling restorative approach. Now she is putting out the invitation to become pregnant. Instead of running, she goes on hikes, using the beauty of nature to remind her of birth happening all around her.

"Poses for men are also important. I teach men asanas that create space in the pelvis, cooling that area, and relaxing the body, such as Baddha Konasana or bound angle pose. Wide leg positions and inversions, Halasana or plow pose, are great. Occasionally I meet a man who has chronically low energy, and then I take a different approach, using active asanas such as tree pose to create more vitality."

Dr. Sethi recommends yoga poses for menstrual pain, and as a mind-body tool. In addition, breathing exercises are used to balance the parasympathetic and sympathetic nervous systems, and she feels that meditation can positively affect Vata. Dr. Patel likes the strengthening effect that yoga has upon the pelvic region, and the way that it increases blood flow and prana. She points out that the philosophy of yoga is also a discipline of mind and body, of surrendering to the universe and to a higher self, as opposed to being in control.

De West describes her own fertility journey and how she used the principles of Ayurveda, yoga, and acupuncture.

I was married for twelve years, but never wanted to have children. It just didn't seem right for that relationship. When I met my second husband, one of the first things he did was to tell me about his nephew, and ask me if I liked kids. It was the first time I thought that maybe I did want children someday.

Our relationship deepened, and at the same time, I was having discomfort in my abdomen that I knew wasn't right. I went to my ob-gyn who did an ultrasound, and it turned out that I had small dermoid cysts on both of my ovaries. At the time, I was thirty-nine. I was so driven to pursue getting pregnant that I opted for a five-hour open abdominal surgery, in which they removed half of each of my ovaries. The surgeon said she didn't know whether the procedure would make me go into menopause.

I did a lot of chanting in bed as I recovered from surgery. A friend of mine gave me a crystal and I held it on my abdomen, visualized healing, and thought, "I have to get pregnant." I did my yoga practice with the intention of healing, went for walks in nature, saw craniosacral practitioners and osteopaths, and worked on restoring my body mentally, physically, and emotionally.

My husband and I got married, and for our honeymoon, we went to India. We spent five weeks there, and every altar or shrine we visited, we asked to have a baby. One temple had an icon of a baby in a crib; you hung it on a tree and said a prayer to Ganesh.

We came back home and started trying to get pregnant. I worked with an acupuncturist who said that I had to tell my body that I'm young, have it release one of those young eggs. At that time I had been vegan for twelve years, and the acupuncturist encouraged me to add some animal protein. I added eggs, took herbs, and did acupuncture, and we got pregnant after a year. Then, I miscarried while teaching a yoga class. I took a couple of months off to deal with that loss and did healing yoga; I was encouraged because at least this proved that I could get pregnant.

It took me another year to get pregnant again. I continued to have acupuncture. After my husband and I made love, I did long inversions. I'd put on a CD of yoga nidra and do a shoulder stand for twenty-five minutes, and then put my legs up on a chair for ten minutes. Then I'd do the Supta Baddha Konasana resting pose. When my period came, I would have a grieving period and let myself cry.

I also added fish into my diet and wound up getting pregnant again. I took very good care of myself; I didn't do active asana or a lot of activity in general. I focused on restorative yoga, walking, and

195

inverting. At thirty-six weeks, I had acupuncture to go into labor, had a natural childbirth in the hospital, and gave birth to my daughter.

Yoga can carry you through loss, celebration, and taking good care of yourself. One of the first tenets of yoga is *ahimsa,* or to do no harm. You try to be in the present moment, do the best you can, and then just be. I believe that yoga is a transformational practice that makes your entire life better.

Do's and Don'ts

1. Don't do a rigorous yoga practice. Too intense a workout can be detrimental to reproductive health. Be gentle with yourself. Do sequences that feel luscious, connecting, and grounding. Move away from more demanding aerobic practices such as Ashtanga or power yoga, toward a more mindful approach to asana.
2. Don't do deep twists if you think there's a chance you could be pregnant. Twists signal the body to squeeze and expel—not the energetics you want to encourage if you are pregnant.
3. Do work on poses that encourage your hips to open and soften; concentrate on postural alignment to ensure that prana flows most efficiently and freely.
4. Do incorporate poses that encourage apana vayu (downward movement of breath), which is employed during reproduction.
5. Do add poses that open up the hips and pelvic area and encourage breath to flow in those areas.
6. Do have some fun with your partner practicing poses together or doing partner poses.

Pranayama

Pranayama, or the breathing exercises of yoga, can be enormously useful in resetting the nervous system. Pranayama can be practiced on its own (some such exercises were described in "Mind-Body Medicine") or used in conjunction with the asanas. Pranayama practices are said to balance the lunar (feminine) and solar (male) channels.

As De West says, "Everyone can benefit from breath awareness. Breath carries you through the asanas with intention. Consciousness comes to your body and mind, and they start to connect."

Linda Sparrowe most often teaches *ujjayi* breath, or "ocean breath" to enhance fertility. To perform ujjayi, first inhale and exhale deeply through the mouth. Then, when exhaling, begin to slightly constrict the flow of air in your throat. In effect, you will be consciously toning the back of your throat and producing a rough, audible sound as you breath out, somewhat reminiscent of crashing waves, and hence the label ocean breath. Once you are comfortable constricting your throat during exhalation, begin to do the same on inhalation. As you master the technique, begin breathing with your mouth closed, through your nose, while continuing to constrict the throat and producing the ujjayi sound.

If you feel tense, Linda recommends *nadi shodana* exercises, or alternate-nostril breathing technique, lengthening the exhalation. In this exercise, you inhale through one nostril, hold the breath, and then exhale through the other nostril. You can practice as follows: Bend the pointer finger and the middle finger of the right hand in toward the palm, keeping the thumb, ring finger, and pinkie finger lifted. Close the right nostril gently with the thumb and inhale fully into the left nostril. Hold the breath without forcing. Close the left nostril with the ring and pinkie fingers, release the right nostril, and exhale completely. Inhale into the right nostril; close the right; open the left and exhale through the left nostril. That constitutes one round of nadi shodhana. Do up to fifteen rounds, stopping at any time if it becomes agitating. Another useful exercise for anxiety and insomnia is *bhramari,* which involves closing the ears and eyes and making a humming sound from the epiglottis in exhale, creating a calming vibration in the head. It is said to help balance the pituitary system and the endocrine system.

For fibroids or endometriosis, there is a special energizing pranayama called *kapal-*

abhati, or "bellows breath." It involves using a forceful breath, which aids Kapha balance. (This is not recommended if you are pregnant.) For this exercise, breathe in and out through your nostrils rapidly, keeping the mouth lightly closed. Inhalation and exhalation should be equal and short, and the action of the chest should be rapid and mechanical. Begin with fifteen seconds and gradually build up to one minute.

Panchakarma

So many of my patients ask me about detoxification. As my colleague Dr. Andrew Weil often says, "The first step to detoxification is to stop taking toxins in." This means making wise choices about our food; environmental chemical exposures; and even, as emphasized in Ayurveda, toxic emotions. In addition, we can amp up the detoxification systems built into our bodies in a variety of ways. We can increase elimination through eating more fiber and drinking plenty of water. Our bodies sweat away toxins, and using a sauna can help us sweat more profusely. Our most sophisticated detoxifying organ is our liver. Liver metabolism can be revved up by eating cruciferous vegetables, and detoxification is aided by taking the herb milk thistle.

Panchakarma is the set of detoxification practices unique to Ayurveda; it is used to bring the doshas into balance, and should be undertaken only under the care of a trained professional. It is recommended when preparing to get pregnant, as well as for infertility issues, since it cleanses the body and mind of any accumulated toxins, thereby creating an optimal state in which to conceive. There are five separate procedures, each of which affects specific doshas. In India, three to four weeks would be set aside to complete this process, during which time a person does not work and allows the mind to rest.

Prior to the detox, people are prepared with an application of medicated oil massage (called oleation, or *snehana*) and then an external application of rice cooked with herbs in a bundle (*swedhana*). An herbal cleansing formula called *triphala* is often used, and the diet is a simple one of rice, lentils, and vegetables, minimizing the work of the digestive system.

The five procedures, which might sound shocking in the twenty-first century, include emesis (vomiting), purgation and enemas, bloodletting, and nasal administration of substances. Not all five are used on every person, as it depends on the doshic imbalance. For some, the preparatory oleation and external application of herbs is sufficient. Emesis is often used for people in whom Kapha is dominant; purgation, for Pitta; and enemas, for Vata. Following the cleanse, agni, or the digestive fire, is rebuilt during a slow resumption of the full diet, normal activities, and yoga and meditation.

Dr. Bhattacharya compares panchakarma to spring-cleaning a room—you need to prepare first by picking up the mess, opening the windows, then doing a thorough job from top to bottom. She says that if you are working twelve hours per day, smoking and drinking, or eating badly, for example, you need to take time to get these residues out of your body before trying to get pregnant. In addition, she recommends that you clear your mind of toxic concerns before conception. Ask yourself if you are too desperate to get pregnant, or if you are trying too hard to make everyone else happy, or dealing with a crazy work schedule. If so, these issues need to be balanced before you try to conceive.

While full panchakarma is not widely available in the United States, Dr. Sethi says that we all can consider doing abyanga for ourselves. This self-massage of the abdomen is traditionally performed with sesame oil in the morning before a bath or shower. Purchase cured organic sesame oil and warm it by running the container under hot water for a few minutes. Dip your fingertips in the oil and apply them lightly to your abdomen. Begin with light, gentle strokes, working the oil into your skin. Move your hands slowly and mindfully in a circular motion in the direction in which the colon empties (clockwise as you look down). Spend several minutes on the practice, and then if you have the time, relax or meditate for the next ten minutes. Then bathe or shower. Done as part of one's morning routine, abyanga is very calming to the nervous system.

Ayurveda and Karma

Ayurveda is rooted in Vedic philosophy, which includes the idea of karma. Everything is thought to play a role in conception, including the mind-set of the parents during intercourse, and even the nostril through which you are breathing (which is said to determine the gender of the baby). In a traditional society, a priest would conduct specific ceremonies, depending on whether the parents desired a boy or a girl. This raises a concern about IVF, which could be seen as changing the nature of things. It is thought that anything done outside of nature could result in some doshic imbalances and possibly unwanted consequences.

The Importance of Ayurveda

Ayurveda brings forth a wisdom generated through thousands of years of careful observation and clinical experience. Long before microscopes and scientific studies, healers were paying exquisite attention to the effects of herbs and dietary and behavioral changes on the body, mind, and spirit. Within Ayurveda, we have the evidence of five thousand years of knowledge gained through trial and error carried down through the generations. Only now are these practices being subjected to randomized clinical trials. While more research studies are needed, we shouldn't discount this other category of evidence born out of five millennia of healers' experience.

CHAPTER 10

SPIRITUALITY

arlier in this book, I discussed readying yourself physically and emotionally for childbirth. Here, I address spiritual preparation. Our spirituality succors us during times of crisis, and its sweet waters also enrich our daily existence. When we think of conceiving a child with joy, we express our gratitude for our own lives and our ability to bear new life. If we are wrestling with infertility, our spiritual resources can help us gain meaning from the experience and surface from the depths of despair.

Spirituality is a deeply personal and intimate realm. Extending beyond religion or dogma, it is where we explore questions of ultimate meaning. It encompasses how we connect to what is sacred, beyond our individual personas. When we talk about spirituality, we are often discussing what really matters to us, and that which gives our lives vitality.

Dr. Rachel Naomi Remen, a pioneer who recognized the role of the spirit in health, the author of *Kitchen Table Wisdom* and one of my teachers, defines spirituality in the following way: "The spiritual . . . is the deepest sense of belonging and participation. We all participate in the spiritual, whether we know it or not. . . .

The most important thing in defining spirit is the recognition that the spirit is an essential need of human nature. There is something in all of us that seeks the spiritual. This yearning varies in strength from person to person, but it is always there in everyone."

People express their spirituality in many different ways. For some, it is through religious practice or faith tradition; for others, it may be communing with nature. While perceived as transcendent—indeed, as some of the most profound moments of our lives—a spiritual experience often loses its power when we try to put it into words. Still, we know what we have felt.

Discussing spirituality can sometimes feel taboo. In my clinical practice, it presents a revealing opportunity to get to know my patients better. I am quite up front about it, asking my patients whether they have religious or faith traditions that are important to them. Some respond with their religion; others describe a faith that they were raised in but no longer practice; still others speak of their connection to nature or a higher power. I delve deeper to learn what spiritual practices, if any, they carry out, inquiring whether they pray, perform rituals, or spend time in nature. When someone tells me, for example, "I'm a recovering Catholic," I ask more about what he may have taken away that holds meaning, and what he has left behind. Depending on my patient's situation, I may ask where she finds strength during challenging times. With others, I question whether they have ever had experiences of awe or mystery, or one they simply cannot explain. These conversations uncover personal values and perspectives that often do not emerge from other topics. They also demand a level of intimacy and trust. And sometimes they reveal profound coping strategies.

Kalpana Shere-Wolfe describes how visualization and prayer impacted her fertility journey. Kalpana had been trying for several years to get pregnant, and eventually, at age thirty-nine, she saw a doctor who said that considering her age, she should go right to IVF. Kalpana did two cycles, but neither worked. At that point, the doctor warned her that her ovaries were not producing enough eggs to harvest, and that he could attempt only one more cycle. "So I had the pressure not only of going through IVF but also hearing the doctor say that my ovaries were 'pooped,'" she commented.

As Kalpana describes it, "Going through the IVF implantation and having it not take felt like I'd lost a baby. On top of the thirty days of shots, the emotional letdown was very hard. But no matter what the doctor said, I told myself, 'No, I'm having a child.' I never gave up hope; the yearning for this child was so deep and strong. I still felt that it was possible, despite my poor prognosis. Yet it was daunting and discouraging to hear the doctor constantly citing statistics that weren't in my favor."

Kalpana used visualization and prayer to remain openhearted, asking the universe and God for a child throughout the third IVF attempt. "There was a lot of outpouring of emotion, and being in touch with how much I wanted to have a baby. It wasn't a happy process like a positive affirmation; instead, I was being honest and letting all of my emotions out in terms of what I truly wanted. In my visualizations, I would see myself, my husband, and a baby, and I'd imagine the things we would do with that baby. I'd let myself feel the emotions as if I was looking down at him in my arms."

During this process, Kalpana also relied upon prayer. Her parents are Hindu, and her husband's parents are from different faith backgrounds. "Growing up in New York, I was surrounded by people of all different religions. I never felt that I was religious per se, but I did feel that I was a spiritual person. My dad allowed us to celebrate every holiday and religion with our friends, so it had less to do with religion and more to do with a spiritual connection to God, a higher being, or the universe."

Kalpana's prayers were not formal; instead, she would sit quietly and let her deep yearning to have a child resonate through her body. "I let those feelings come up, and it was my way of speaking to God or the universe. I allowed my love and desire for a child to be my prayer in my quiet moments alone. It never left my consciousness."

With her third IVF attempt, Kalpana produced two eggs, and both embryos implanted. The odds of this happening were so low that she felt it was a miracle. Before she knew there were two embryos, she lost one, yet she still felt that she was having a baby. She later found out that the other embryo was still in place.

Given her age, Kalpana was offered amniocentesis, but she declined any tests because she was 100 percent sure this child was for her, whether he was healthy or not. "I felt that even if there were problems, this baby would be the perfect child for me; that was my mind-set. I tapped into it inside myself that this was going to happen; it didn't matter what the doctor said. I never gave in to believing that it wasn't possible; I never gave up on having a child. Believing in a miracle made it easier to go through IVF, and finding positive feelings within myself made a huge difference."

Kalpana and her husband went on to have a healthy son, whom they named Kiran. "We feel that he is a gift from the universe," she says.

Kalpana didn't have a support group while going through this difficult process, so she tries to share her story whenever she feels it could help someone. Once when she returned to her fertility doctor's office with Kiran, she saw a despondent-looking woman in the waiting room and was moved to tell her about her own experience. A year later she ran into the same woman at the city zoo, pushing twin babies in a stroller.

Kalpana sums up her experience this way: "My path was following my own intuition from moment to moment, to try to make everything more positive. You can't put yourself in a happy mind-set in this situation, but I tried to have a strong belief that it was possible for me to have a child." Kalpana feels that having an established yoga and spiritual practice helped her when going through IVF because it built on the foundation of who she is as a fundamentally spiritual person. "I couldn't have been so unwavering in my belief that I'd have a baby, without the foundation of those practices, because they take me back to nature, and my belief in a higher power. Ask openly with your heart, and what you seek, you shall receive."

In my personal life, I have found great meaning in religious ritual and spiritual ceremonies. While I have learned many traditional prayers, often, when I pray, I find myself simply speaking from my heart. In addition to the practices of my own faith, I have participated in Native American purification lodges, immersion in healing waters, Buddhist meditation, and Sanskrit chants. These practices serve as vehicles to ask for guidance during times of difficulty. They help me reframe suffering as not just a terrible experience, but also as something with a larger meaning from which I might grow. They help me to be centered, and they remind me that all is not under my control.

I hope that you will spend some time pondering the mystery of birth. What does it mean to you to create a new life? Do you believe there is a way in which you can send out a welcoming message to a new soul? What does it mean to you to prepare to receive? Can you "conceive" of yourself as the vessel from which life will emerge?

Whether or not you relate to the idea of a soul, there is much to conception and birth that reminds us of everyday miracles—how from the biological union of egg and sperm, this unique child is born to these two parents. When you consider pregnancy in this way, you may be intrigued by the possibility of preparing yourself spiritually with ceremony or prayer. Indeed, in the world of mysticism, birth is considered one of the great feminine initiations.

In this chapter, I explore a spectrum of practices, from secular spirituality to the role of ceremony and ritual and the teachings of common religions. Find what resonates with your belief system and consider developing a spiritual practice if you do not have one already.

Conducting a Ceremony

Consider a wedding ceremony. It usually includes deciding whom to invite, choosing a place, selecting a religious leader or justice of the peace to conduct the service, and picking a honeymoon destination. It also includes rituals, or symbolic activities, that are embedded into the larger ceremony. A wedding can include cherished traditions such as the exchange of rings, the sharing of vows, and the reading of scripture or blessings. And at times, couples make up new, deeply personal rituals to mark the event.

Like getting married, having a child is a passage after which you will be alive in the world in a new way. As you consider this major milestone that involves crossing a threshold from being an adult without children to becoming a parent, you can choose to consciously mark the transition. A ceremony is one way to do this, and it can help you prepare emotionally and spiritually for this next phase of life.

For example, having a baby will impact many of your relationships. You not only become a parent, but also turn your parents into grandparents, and your siblings into aunts and uncles. Your relationship with your spouse is likely to be altered—with the baby becoming your number-one priority and your spouse moving into second place. You become vulnerable in the world in a way that is both life-affirming and frightening. Suddenly you are responsible for the life of another being.

All transitions involve gains and losses. Ceremony gives you the opportunity to sanctify what you are moving toward in an intentional way. With the birth of a child, you experience the miracle of a new baby, the profound love that emerges, and the joy of your own parents. At the very same time, you experience serious sleep deprivation, the loss of the primacy of your marital relationship, and reduced freedom to move about the world with ease and spontaneity.

Rituals symbolically express these changes. They help us move from one state of awareness to another. They do so by allowing us to transcend our personal experience and to connect with all the men and women before us who have borne children, given up the carefree attitude of young adulthood, and gained the mantle of parenthood. Rituals can help us move beyond our rational, thinking, even skeptical minds and open us to new possibilities. They help us gain awareness of inner resources; think of the ferocious love a mother carries for her child.

Developing a ceremony to prepare for conception can be approached in many different ways. You can build upon known rituals, such as using a family priest and a traditional ceremony; you may decide to adapt an established tradition to fit your own purpose; or you can create a ceremony that is entirely new. The mood for your ceremony can be celebratory or serious, personal or public; you can do it alone or with your partner, or invite your full community.

A fertility ceremony can include gift giving, a reading or a poem, reciting the history of your family lineage, or using a guided visualization. You can perform rituals such as an immersion or anointing with water or oil. You may want to frame some questions about what you wish to leave behind, things to recall and take with you from the past, or things to create anew for the future. Developing a ceremony is creative and serves as a modern expression of spirituality that connects you to the new life ahead.

One traditional Jewish ritual to prepare for conception is the *mikveh*. Observant women immerse themselves in a deep, indoor pool of rainwater before marriage and after each menstrual period, before recommencing sexual relations with their husbands. It is said that when women enter the mikveh, they enter the realm of the divine, for the waters of the mikveh are drawn from the heavens.

"Ceremony is a way of connecting to something larger, but also to the subconscious. Our minds have no idea about many things that go on in our bodies. Ceremony is a way that we can drop into ourselves in a manner that we aren't capable of doing through ordinary awareness," says Ann Marie Chiasson, MD, a family physician with training in energy medicine who is on the faculty at the Arizona Center for Integrative Medicine. She teaches meditation and develops ceremonies for the center's Fellows as well as for others.

Across different cultures, ceremonies are often structured in similar ways because they are wired into the psyche. It is as if we are following an invisible map into deeper layers for healing. From a Jungian perspective, we are jumping into the unconscious; a Shamanic or indigenous model would describe it as connecting to our ancestors or to nature. In any case, we are accessing something beyond the ordinary. Dr. Chiasson points out that "Humans have been doing fertility rituals since the beginning of time, since nature was the first god and fertility was the initial impulse in asking for rain, crops, and animals to hunt."

Howard Silverman, MD, coauthor with Carl Hammerschlag of *Healing Ceremonies,* says, "Ceremonies create times of blessing; ceremonies provide a structure for getting in touch with our hearts; ceremonies help us see old certainties in a new way."

Over the years, Dr. Silverman has helped many people develop all kinds of personal ceremonies, ranging from one he did with his wife to help them and their family come to terms with their daughter's congenital blindness, to marriage ceremonies. He has developed a rich set of ideas over the years about the process of creating a ceremony.

"Conducting a ceremony has two intrinsic purposes: reinforcing one's social network, and increasing the perception of control," Dr. Silverman says. He outlines seven steps to creating the event: articulating a shared purpose, shared preparation, identifying the community and the facilitator, establishing the opening, using shared symbolic processes, using ceremonial objects (particularly those which affect the senses), and the closing.

Initially, you publicly state your purpose: what you want to have happen. You must be able to explain it to others in just a few sentences. For example: "We are beginning to prepare for a new stage in our lives, and we wish to do it consciously and thoughtfully. We want to open ourselves to becoming parents." Or you could say, "We ask you to join together with us as we create an opening in our family and community for a new life." To "celebrate" means to share publicly; creating a celebration of conception announces your desire to receive a child.

Next, decide who the attendees should be. You could include your parents, friends, and a spiritual advisor, or it could be just you and your partner. Some people want their parents to attend, while others do not. Invite the people in your life to whom you'd look for support, those who will understand your intentions and with whom you feel safe.

The opening can involve a reading, the lighting of a candle or a fire, music, or other creative options. It should indicate that people can let themselves fully enter the ceremony. Often participants go into a light trance where they lose track of time as they become entirely focused on the present moment. Later they might comment, "Two hours went by? It felt as if we were here for two minutes."

The ceremony itself is limited only by your imagination. Almost all involve a transition and an exposition of what is being lost and what gained. Rather than multiple steps, keep the ceremony focused on the purpose; the simpler, the better.

In one workshop that Dr. Silverman conducted, each person created an item and talked to the group about the meaning it held for them. One woman made a pouch with bells in it, symbolizing the child she wanted to have. It became a very potent symbol for her. Rituals are not formulaic; what works as a symbol for one person might not hold true for another.

A clear-cut closing gives people a feeling of safety, wherein they can emerge from the experience. This can occur in any number of ways; ideally, it is a gentle transition back to ordinary reality. Symmetry works well for closing; for example, lighting and then extinguishing a candle, or offering a reading at the beginning and end. This signals that that which was opened is now closed, and provides balance for the whole experience.

Dr. Chiasson agrees that simplicity is a plus. "A ceremony requires a beginning, middle, and end. The opening can be as simple as going outside, or lighting a candle. You can be alone, or be with someone else. The middle can be whatever comes to you, such as bleeding into the earth or putting your hands on your belly; then you should create an ending. Some people make it far too complicated, involving multiple steps, and moving from one activity to the next. Hold the ceremony as something quite sacred. And you can take this new mystical awareness into lovemaking, having blood tests, or medical intervention such as IVF."

The energetic level in ceremony, says Dr. Chiasson, is a way for a woman to move into a visceral connection to the world around her. We realize that we are not disconnected from all other women having children, or from the cycles of nature. Our fertility is in synch; women menstruate together, and there is a larger energy field that we're all in touch with. The ceremony allows women to access that connection. When people move into a ceremonial space, they can hear things in a new way and listen to their bodies differently than when using rational thought. It's the difference between walking around thinking about something and having a gut feeling.

Dr. Chiasson described her own fertility ceremony: "When I was ready to get pregnant with my first child, I went into a meditation and visualized myself dropping down into my body. I landed on top of my uterus, and I asked, what should I do? What came to me was that I needed to go outside when I was having my next period, and bleed into the earth. I went out at night in my bathrobe, dug a hole, bled into the earth, and covered it over. In that ceremony, I realized that my body wasn't mine, that I was connected to something much deeper, and my blood actually belonged to the earth. As it turned out, my actions were very similar to ancient rituals that women have done over time and in many cultures. The ancient Celtic ritual of Beltane (or May day) was one such fertility rite.

"On an energy level, it was the first time my root chakra opened and was able to stay open enough to have children. The root chakra is the first chakra, and it is the energy center in the body that relates to reproduction. The two chakras most involved in fertility are the root chakra and the second chakra, or in TCM, the lower Dan-Tian. Most people approach having a baby from their minds, but energetically, it is about having the chakras open. This is why yoga and TCM work; once these chakras are opened, the rest of it takes care of itself."

The process of ceremony involves talking truthfully and symbolically. As you prepare for the occasion, gather materials such as clothing and objects that have been passed along in your family, which can serve as symbols of your purpose. Old things, such as a great-grandmother's brooch or objects that have been used frequently in a ceremonial context, have intrinsic power. Often it's in the preparation, when you are gathering your materials and thinking of your loss and gain, that the healing occurs. For instance, a woman who miscarried late and was unable to let go of her grief had the idea of planting three beautiful flowering plants. She chose two perennials, to represent the children that she had, and one annual, which she knew would die at the end of the season, to represent the baby who had died. She tended the flowers carefully, and was surprised to feel when the annual died that it seemed part of the natural cycle of things. In her preparation, she had integrated her loss.

Some women adopt rituals that build on the metaphor of planting seeds. In conception, we are opening ourselves to whatever children the universe sends. This can be symbolically enacted by taking a bunch of seeds, mixing them up, planting them, and watching to see what grows.

You can express your vision of conception using any of your senses: painting an abstract picture, drumming, lighting a candle, or performing a religious rite.

A feeling of social connectedness can result from performing a ceremony. This can be particularly sweet if you have felt disconnected because you have not yet been able to conceive. You may find that you can move from a sense of isolation, or jealousy that everyone but you is having babies. Instead of the secrecy that often surrounds trying to get pregnant, you can build a sense of community, articulate some of your angst, and feel reconnected. The comfort derived from expressing your feelings with this trusted group of people in a safe space can be profound. At best, it provides the sense that you are not just at the mercy of the universe, that there is a larger framework. A formal ceremony, witnessed by other people, can also be used to adjust to not being able to conceive. In speaking directly and truthfully, you may also articulate a different vision about pregnancy; for instance, realizing that there are other ways to funnel the desire for a child, such as mentoring or adoption.

A colleague of mine told me the following story about a ceremony that she performed after enduring several miscarriages.

>I was early in my fourth pregnancy, having lost three pregnancies beforehand. After my third miscarriage and before conceiving for the fourth time, both my husband and I wrote a letter to the other babies we had lost, and invited the new soul to come in. Returning from a spiritual retreat in Hawaii, a friend who had studied energy medicine and Kabbalah did a long-distance healing. She felt that there was a male soul trying to come through.

>I became pregnant after that healing; my conception was announced to me in a dream before I missed my period.

>My husband and I had planned to attend another weeklong retreat in Hawaii with a dear teacher and some close friends. It was week six of the fourth pregnancy, and I had started spotting, which was the norm for me. We decided to go to the retreat, and not to let the fear of losing another pregnancy deter us.

>Upon arriving in Hawaii, I continued to spot slightly, and my breasts were not as tender. I feared another loss. On the fifth day of

the retreat, our teacher asked me if I would be open to a ceremony, and I said yes. Knowing how reserved I am, he offered either to do it in private with just a couple of people, or else with the whole attending community of around twenty people. I replied that I was fine with the whole group.

My husband and I first spoke of our ancestors and their tribulations. Then, our teacher created what he called a "grief basket" for me. I lay on a blanket and was covered with another blanket. Then, he chose a few women to surround me and hold me. An elderly woman held my womb; another woman, my feet; while connecting to Krishna through Sarada Devi, a Bengali Holy Mother. Another woman breathed kindness, and two other women held my heart. The group chanted: "Where are you, my son; where are you, my daughter . . ." a made-up song. My husband got spontaneous support from three men in the group.

I found myself releasing grief, and sending love to all the babies that had tried to come through me. I remember thinking that all that I had to do was to give love; to love those I had not loved yet, and to give more love to those I had already loved. I felt tremendous peace and surrender; it was very healing. At the end of the ceremony, many in the room were sobbing. Our teacher said: "When one heart shatters, many others are healed."

Although I still felt grief, I also felt healed. On returning to the continental United States, I went to my scheduled appointment with the ob-gyn. A fetal heart was seen on an ultrasound. I was surprised and thrilled.

The Religious Perspective

In many religions, as in mythology, a man's path to God involves a journey. On the other hand, Biblical women often deepen their connection to God through the experience of infertility. Hannah's tale from the Old Testament book of Samuel reveals how she became an example of fervent prayer. Hannah was absolutely clear about what she wanted—pleading for a child, and pledging her son to God.

According to the story, Hannah wanted a child, but for years was unable to conceive. She desired a pregnancy so much that at one point, her husband asked, "Am I not enough for you?" Yet she never stopped praying for a baby. One year she made a pilgrimage to the Temple in Jerusalem with her family. The high priest, Eli, witnessed her praying and chastised her for being drunk because he saw "her lips were constantly moving, yet no sound issued forth." Hannah's prayer was, "O Lord of Hosts, if You will look upon the suffering of Your maidservant and will remember me and not forget Your maidservant, and if You will grant Your maidservant a male child, I will dedicate him to the Lord for all the days of his life" (1 Samuel 1:11). Eventually her prayer was granted, and she conceived and had her longed-for infant.

Hannah's story captures something of the complexity of human prayer. Prayer offers us the opportunity to turn our hearts' deepest yearnings into words. We put our hearts on the line, even bargain away things that we cannot deliver—prayer answered or not—when crying out in the most raw, genuine way imaginable. In so doing, we discover something about ourselves. We learn what we're willing to stake our lives for.

At times, we desire something so passionately that we make specific requests and, like Hannah, even try to strike bargains with God. Religion can give us a larger context to hold our longings and at times our losses. We can make prayers of petition, and every religion has such prayers for a child. We can surrender ourselves to "God's will." We can hold difficulty conceiving as being "tested" by God. Some couples consider infertility to be a punishment from God. All of these religious perspectives appear among us—some more consciously than others. Yet, all of us acknowledge that having a baby is beyond human power. We can prepare in every possible way and make ourselves vessels, but the creation of life is ultimately not up to us.

A Catholic friend described the role that prayer played in her attempt to conceive. At age thirty-nine, she had had two miscarriages. She and her husband hadn't told anyone else that she was pregnant, and they kept the miscarriages to themselves. However, the third time she got pregnant, the couple asked everyone close to them to pray for her. When my friend told her mother about the miscarriages, her mother revealed that she herself had had two miscarriages, and had never told anyone. This revelation helped my friend deal with her loss, and thankfully her third pregnancy resulted in the birth of long-awaited twin boys.

Every major religion includes prayers for a child. The prayers of one's youth, which connect deeply into one's heritage, can be a source of comfort and strength. More general prayers such as the Lord's prayer, attributed to Jesus, and simply phrased as "thy will be done," may speak to your heart. Abraham Joshua Heschel writes in *Man's Quest for God,* "To pray is to take notice of the wonder, to regain a sense of the mystery that animates all beings, the divine margin in all attainments." Please see "Additional Resources" for some examples of fertility prayers. Consider reciting one from your own lineage, or creating a prayer of your own.

Religion can be an incredible source of coping. Faith, traditions, and beliefs can be a source of strength during difficult times. We can find spiritual support from a minister, priest, rabbi, an imam, or in a congregation. By engaging in religious activities, we can shift our focus away from our personal trials to help others. In addition, we can redefine infertility as a test that leads to acceptance and spiritual growth.

Unfortunately, for others, religion can be a source of added pain. Some people experience infertility as God's punishment and rail against God. Infertility becomes a negative experience of religion. The feeling is, why did he give everyone else a child, but not me? In this way, religion can be a source of further crisis. When this happens, some people wholeheartedly reject the religion of their birth. In my practice, when I encounter this reaction, I may suggest a session with a religious leader, a spiritual director, or a therapist, in order to work through these feelings.

A spiritual counselor can help us sort out how we make sense of adversity, and what to do with our disappointment. I have often remembered, during difficult times, Kierkegaard's words: "Life must be lived forward, but can only be understood backward." When life doesn't go the way we had hoped, we can sometimes make sense of the setbacks through a spiritual or religious connection. We can seek to find meaning in loss. When we do, this can be transformative.

Religion and Fertility

Beginning with the Old Testament, and forming a central injunction of many religions, God commands us to "be fruitful and multiply," yet religious leaders have varying interpretations of modern medical fertility technologies. Christian churches such as the Church of England and the Baptist, Episcopal, Methodist, and Mennonite churches have liberal attitudes toward IVF with spouse gametes, as long as there is no embryo wastage. Judaism allows all techniques of assisted reproduction when the egg and sperm belong to the wife and husband. Some rabbinical authorities reject donor eggs; others permit them, as long as the husband assents. The Vatican is morally opposed to IVF, as well as to artificial insemination by a donor, or by a husband when the semen is collected by masturbation. It also opposes embryo freezing and surrogate motherhood; only interfallopian transfer is acceptable. Islam allows reproductive technology if the sperm and egg are from the husband and wife, and the resulting embryo is transferred to the wife's uterus. Third-party involvement is not acceptable.

Occasionally our religious beliefs can conflict with our efforts to conceive. Ilana and Neil Markowitz live in Tucson, and participated in the Modern Orthodox Jewish community there. At age thirty-three, Ilana, a yoga teacher, was starting to think about having a child. She and her husband were following the Jewish laws of family purity regarding rules for marital relations. This ancient practice involves refraining from intercourse for a minimum of twelve days, beginning with the first day of a woman's period, and concluding with a mikveh, or ritual bath.

Ilana loved the ritual and holiness of the practice, but ran into a significant problem. Because she had always had a short cycle, she found herself ovulating on day 10–11. This meant that she and Neil were not allowed to have intercourse on the days that she was actually fertile. She felt anxious and sad about having to choose between following the ritual laws and having a child. After more than a year, she stopped following the ritual; then she and Neil attempted to conceive for an ensuing year. She felt that she had somehow taken in the message that "something is wrong with my body." This, unfortunately, was reinforced when she saw a fertility doctor. He prescribed Clomid, which didn't help, then followed it with four months of injec- 215 tions, but she did not become pregnant. During this time her stepsister conceived by accident, which was emotionally difficult for Ilana.

Then Ilana happened to see John Friend, the yoga teacher who founded Anusara, at a workshop he was teaching. (Anusara is a form of hatha yoga in which the foundational principle is opening to grace.) John agreed to consult with Ilana about her fertility challenges. He conveyed confidence that through the practice's energy and attitude of grace, he could help her to conceive. He taught her specific yoga postures, the main orientation of which was unlocking the openings of the reproductive area. John advised Ilana, "You need to open your sails to catch the winds of grace."

Ilana also saw a traditional Chinese medicine practitioner who was pregnant at the time. In addition to acupuncture, she gave Ilana an herbal mixture with thirty-two ingredients, which she was instructed to steep on the stove in a glass pot. Ilana also read a thesis from a rabbinical program that discussed Jewish traditional paths for personal development. She was intrigued to learn that there was a gender difference. For men, what was typically conveyed in the biblical stories was a "hero's journey" of leaving one's home and finding a connection to God in a new place. For women, connection often took place as women underwent the test of infertility and its resolution. This treatise gave Ilana a sense that there was something positive in her fertility struggle.

Ilana felt that John's and her acupuncturist's belief that they could help her was instrumental in relieving her anxiety. As Ilana puts it, "Surrender was key. I had been trying to make something happen that was beyond my own will, but now I felt like I could share the responsibility. They had experience and confidence, because they'd had results before with other patients. I didn't feel that way with the fertility doctors who simply recited statistics; from them I only sensed pessimism, and felt no sense of partnership."

She and Neil also went to see David Rubenstein, a Kabbalistic astrologer in Phoenix. He gave them a fertility astrology reading, working up their charts by hand. David told them that there was a window of time when they would be most fertile together. Rubenstein also mentioned that after conceiving and having a baby, the window would remain wide-open, and to be careful because they could quickly conceive again.

All of this helped Ilana reconsider her belief that something was wrong with her body. Instead, she began to feel that she had experienced a rite of passage. She reframed the years of struggle as time spent tuning up her body, and she let go of the idea that there was something wrong with her.

After using acupuncture and herbs for seven months, Ilana conceived. Her son, Zakkai, was born when she was thirty-seven. Nine months after Zakkai was born, she got pregnant again, and then her daughter, Aliya, was born.

As a yoga teacher, Ilana shares her story with women who are having fertility issues. She teaches the specific yoga poses that John Friend taught her, and provides the message of being open to grace.

Prayer and the Relaxation Response

Prayer can also be used, as described in the mind-body medicine chapter, to elicit the relaxation response. A large body of evidence on the positive value of prayer shows that when people use rosaries or recite traditional prayers, physiological benefits can result, literally calming the nervous system.

Even if you are not religious, you may find comfort in prayer, the attempt to speak the unspeakable. Quietly or aloud, you can struggle to put into words all that is in your heart. In the opening of this chapter, Kalpana Shere-Wolfe didn't recite a specific prayer; she simply held an intention. This is one way to pray. Another is beautifully expressed in a poem titled *Praying* by Pulitzer prize–winning poet Mary Oliver:

It doesn't have to be
the blue iris, it could be
weeds in a vacant lot, or a few
small stones; just
pay attention, then patch

a few words together and don't try

to make them elaborate, this isn't
a contest but the doorway

into thanks, and a silence in which
another voice may speak.

Speaking from the depths of your heart is the first step in prayer. For most of us, listening for a response is even more challenging. Often it comes as an inner knowing, a clarity of what is called for in this moment. And when we have this experience, we know it to be true. We sense a timeless wisdom. Or as Heschel says, "Prayer takes the mind out of the narrowness of self-interest and enables us to see the world in the mirror of the holy."

Developing a Sense of Gratitude

Adversity can lead us to a greater sense of meaning, and challenges us to live in accord with our values. Often, coming to an understanding of events includes developing a sense of gratitude for all that we have.

A friend of mine had a child who was stillborn, and then went on to have a second child. Her marriage ended, and my friend believes that if her first child had survived, she wouldn't have had her second child because the marriage didn't survive the stress of parenthood. She is grateful for how things worked out, because she cannot imagine life without her son.

After eight miscarriages, including two IVF pregnancies that ended in loss, another friend and her husband decided to adopt. She says that she truly is glad that none of those pregnancies worked out, because if they had, she would not have her little girl. She and her husband feel that their daughter is without a doubt the child they were meant to have, and that she is the ideal person to complete their family, having brought so much joy into their lives.

Mythology and Fertility Goddesses

We have all seen fertility icons from older civilizations; these primitive statues typically feature abundant breasts, large hips, and pregnant bellies. While traveling in Ireland, I was given a Sheela-na-gig carving. Such figures are found in medieval churches and castles all over the country. Featuring widely spread legs and prominent vulvas and vaginal openings, they appear sexually outrageous. Demonstrating Sheela's widespread integration into the culture, she has survived beyond pagan times in strictly Catholic Ireland to the modern day, as church leaders cast a blind eye when women prayed to her image under the light of a full moon.

Almost every primitive culture on earth has at least one fertility goddess, and the stories surrounding them are fascinating. For instance, the Greek goddess associated with fertility is Persephone, daughter of Demeter, the harvest goddess. As the myth goes, one day the young maiden Persephone was out gathering flowers, and the earth below her split in two. Hades, god of the underworld, came charging up in his chariot and kidnapped Persephone.

Demeter searched the ends of the world for her daughter, neglecting her duties. The earth became barren. Finally, with the help of the goddess Hecate, she located Persephone and successfully negotiated with the gods to bring her back. Persephone, who longed to see her mother again, accepted six pomegranate seeds from Hades upon hearing she would be freed. These few morsels sealed her fate; while she could visit the earth for six months every year, initiating the months of spring and summer, when the earth blooms and plants grow, she would have to return underground during the fall and winter.

An Athenian fertility ritual recognizing Persephone took place each September. For nine days women fasted, then purified themselves by bathing in the ocean and walking to the temple in Eleusis, some hours away. They entered the temple, were led through a maze, and shown a sheaf of grain to symbolize the fruitfulness of the fields. Upon leaving the temple, the women broke their fasts with a drink of water mixed with mint and meal.

Throughout antiquity, the natural world heralds similar fertility goddesses and rituals. In Egypt, frogs were seen as symbols of fertility; in Native American tribes, the corn maiden is a potent fertility figure. The many kernels in corn and the seeds of a pomegranate represent abundance and, by extension, reproduction.

While we may no longer pray to goddesses for conception, instinctively we recognize the larger mystery in conception. Take the time to contemplate the spiritual role that you play in the creation of a new life. Mysticism teaches us that there are three partners in creation: a woman, a man, and God. What might you do to draw forth the participation of this triad?

THE PAST AND THE FUTURE

A woman envies her sister, who has had many children with ease. She cannot conceive, although she has tried everything. In desperation, she convinces her husband to use a surrogate, who bears a child for her. Not long after that, she conceives on her own.

Does this sound like a tale from your daily newspaper? Actually it is the biblical story of Jacob and his wives, Rachel and Leah. Leah had six sons with Jacob, but Rachel had yet to conceive. Miserable in her infertility, and longing for a child, Rachel gave her maidservant Bilhah to Jacob. Soon after, Bilhah gave birth "upon Rachel's knees," serving as an early model of a surrogate mother. Rachel's story is yet another that reveals the primal longing for a child.

From time immemorial, having children has been considered a birthright and a blessing. Happily, most adults' longing for a child is achieved with ease. To up the odds that conception comes easily and that your baby is born healthy, I have recommended that you prepare your body, mind, and spirit.

Think back to the principles of integrative medicine and put them into action: Find a physician who feels like a true partner as you embark on your fertility journey.

Pay close attention to the factors that influence your health and wellness, and take steps to be as healthy as you possibly can. If your diet is awry, correct it. If you are under stress, develop a mind-body practice. If you need to drop some weight, lose it. Learn to reduce exposure to environmental toxins that disrupt your hormonal system.

Begin with a self-assessment and evaluate your body, as well as your mind and heart. Do you have habits that might be working against your fertility? Ask yourself, how can I change? Some women make many changes at once; others begin with a single step and go more slowly. Some find that having a partner or asking others to hold them accountable for their health makes all the difference. Reconsider striving, as opposed to receiving. Look deep into your heart to see whether it is necessary for you to carry a pregnancy yourself, or whether adoption might do. Ask what you need to do to conceive, and listen carefully. Consider what it means to ready yourself to receive life. To become a vessel for a baby to grow and develop is to hold the mystery of birth in a spiritual context.

Then if you must do IVF, you will be more likely to be successful as a result of your lifestyle changes. In 2010, a study revealed that women adhering to the Mediterranean diet had better IVF outcomes than those following a health-conscious, low-processed-food diet. Alice Domar's 2011 study showed that women in the mind-body groups conceived more easily with IVF than those not participating in the sessions. The call to be as healthy as possible may help you to conceive naturally, and it has been proven to enhance success with IVF.

Choose carefully among the conventional and alternative options available to you. While recognizing the incredible advances of modern fertility treatment, ranging from hormones, to IVF, to donor sperm and eggs, to surrogacy, you may not want to resort to high-tech measures right away. Instead begin with more natural and less invasive interventions to avoid the risks inherent in these treatments.

At the same time, be discerning when alternative medicine promises to cure all, and turn to conventional medicine when you've reached the limits of lifestyle change. Be prevention oriented, and factor in your age as you consider parenthood; for women, our biology has set fertility highest in our twenties, with dramatic declines after the age of thirty-five. Expect your doctor to walk the talk and to be an open-minded skeptic, willing to consider possibilities outside the scope of Western medical training.

Pioneering research points to another reason to attend to lifestyle issues: the effect they have on future generations. Epigenetics reveals ways in which diet, exercise, and reducing your exposure to environmental toxins affects not only you but also your child, and possibly your grandchildren and great-grandchildren. A growing body of epigenetic research affirms the overwhelming influence of lifestyle on how your genetic code, as laid out by your DNA, is actually expressed. Optimizing your health before conception serves the generations that follow, and may have a lasting influence on many lives to come.

If this book has spurred outrage about the unhealthy diet, high stress, and environmental chemicals that we are exposed to daily, consider becoming an activist. Yes, the corporations are large and powerful, but Margaret Mead's famous quote bears repeating here: "Never doubt that a small group of thoughtful, committed citizens can change the world; indeed, it is the only thing that ever has." Similarly worth advocating for is societal change that would support men and women bearing children at younger ages, so that fewer advanced reproductive technologies are needed. While the biological time clock is particularly sensitive in women, the evidence that older fathers have children with higher rates of autism, lower IQs, and more schizophrenia continues to grow. There are many groups working to promote change in our culture that would welcome your efforts.

If you are having difficulty in getting pregnant, diligently following the suggestions presented in this book may well tip the balance in your favor. Though we live in modern times, we can still turn to prayer and to ritual. Think about obtaining a traditional Chinese medicine assessment and having acupuncture treatments. The ability to conceive may improve when a shift of mind occurs, as evidenced by some of the stories in this book. Many of the women who shared their stories did so to inspire and provide hope to others; although told that their situations were difficult, they persevered and had babies. Please write me at victoria@victoriamaizesmd.com with your stories as well.

In closing, I wish you the blessing of fertility. May you become pregnant with ease; may you carry that pregnancy to term and bear a healthy child; and may that child bring you all the joys of parenthood.

ACKNOWLEDGMENTS

While many describe writing a book as a solo act, I was fortunate enough to have a village of support. I am deeply indebted to many incredible colleagues and friends who stepped forward to share their wisdom, experience, and stories about fertility. I am especially grateful to the wonderful fellows and faculty of the Arizona Center for Integrative Medicine, who gave so generously of their time and expertise. I am deeply moved by the women and men who told intimate, and sometimes private, stories of their journeys to parenthood, in order to serve as beacons of hope and to inspire others to find a passage to fertility.

There are some dear colleagues and friends whom I must mention specifically. Leslie Wells, an amazing collaborator, whose skillful writing and editing helped move this book from an idea into a tangible and readable reality. My sister, Rachel Maizes, a gifted writer and editor, gave invaluable advice on some of the more challenging chapters. Devorah Coryell read and reread multiple versions, shared her wisdom, and was always encouraging. Tara Lemmey tirelessly reviewed chapters and gave me feedback about whether the text carried "my voice." Dr. Ann Marie Chiasson patiently listened as I talked about fertility week after week on our hikes in Sabino Canyon; she also added her wisdom about ceremony and the energetics of fertility. Dr. Si Reichlin reviewed the entire manuscript with scientific rigor and an adept eye for any inconsistencies in writing style.

Very special thanks to my agent, Richard Pine, who believed in me from day one; and to Whitney Frick, my editor, who envisioned the need for a book that guided women to proactively prepare for pregnancy. I couldn't have asked for a better team!

I deeply appreciate the valuable interviews with fellows and graduates of the Arizona Center for Integrative Medicine, including Adi Benito, M.D.; Kevin Coughlin, M.D.; Michele Couri, M.D.; Nathan Daley, M.D.; Julianne Garrison, M.D.; Claudia Harsh, M.D.; Angela LaSalle, M.D.; Ta Ya Lee, N.P.; Joanne Perron, M.D.; Barbi Phelps-Sandall, M.D.; Tanmeet Sethi, M.D.; Carmelo Sgarlata, M.D.; Kalpana Shere-Wolfe, M.D.; and Jingduan Yang, M.D. Their knowledge and perspective enriched these pages.

Integrative medicine experts from around the country who were extremely generous in granting me time for interviews include Helen Adrienne, M.S.W.; Mary Beth Augustine, R.D.; Judith Balk, M.D.; Bhaswati Bhattacharya, M.D.; Tracy Crane, M.S., R.D.; Alice Domar, Ph.D.; Ilana Markowitz, M.S.W.; Leslie McGee, R.N. LAc.; Maggie Ney, N.D.; Sharyle Patton; Premal Patel, M.D.; Howard Silverman, M.D.; Linda Sparrowe; David Wallinga, M.D.; and De West. You will find their wisdom woven through the chapters.

To the faculty and staff at the Arizona Center for Integrative Medicine, I owe the deepest gratitude. To Andrew Weil, M.D., for your mentorship: I believe it was you who inducted me into the art of writing. Thank you for enthusiastic support of the project and for your wonderful foreword. Tieraona Low Dog, M.D., was my first writing partner and co-editor of *Integrative Women's Health*; I miss our "book club" and honor your knowledge and spirit, which found their way into these pages. My assistant, Darlene Kerr, who provided incredible logistical support by tirelessly printing hundreds of articles and setting up all of my interviews. Randy Horwitz, M.D., Ph.D.; Patricia Lebensohn, M.D.; Sally Dodds, Ph.D.; Hilary McClafferty, M.D.; Rubin Naimin, Ph.D.; and Steven Gurgevich, Ph.D., my incredible colleagues at the Center: I have learned from each of you, and so you, too, are reflected in this work.

In addition, I would like to acknowledge the gift of mentorship and the many other teachers who have helped me on my journey, among them Dana Davies, Diane

Katz, Sharon Keating, Nicholas Rango, Rachel Naomi Remen, Hal Williamson, and Jon Kabat-Zinn—thank you.

Finally, my profound gratitude to my parents, Hannah (of blessed memory) and Isaac Maizes, who brought me into this world and had faith in me, and to my wonderful children, Gabrielle, Aaron, and Zoe, who taught me the true blessing of fertility.

ADDITIONAL RESOURCES

Chapter 1: Integrative Medicine Assessment
Web site that describes the principles of integrative medicine: http://www.integrativemedi-
    cine.arizona.edu

Chapter 2: Your Body, Your Lifestyle, and Fertility
BMI calculator: http://www.nhlbisupport.com/bmi/

Chapter 3: Nutrition
Check local dairies, eggs, and infant formula: http://www.cornucopia.org
Web site about calorie intake: http://www.livestrong.com/article/264438-how-many-calo-
    ries-should-a-woman-eat-per-day-to-lose-weight/
Dirty Dozen and Clean Fifteen: http://www.ewg.org
Web site about healthy nutrition: http://www.eatwellguide.org
Web site about healthy foods: http://www.healthyfoodinhealthcare.org
Web site about the new food pyramid: http://www.choosemyplate.gov
Web site about mercury levels in fish: http://www.blueocean.org. The Blue Ocean Institute
    keeps a comprehensive list of fish and their levels of mercury and/or PCBs. Alternatively,
    you can text the word "fish" (followed by the type of fish) to 30644, and they will text

you back. Play close attention, as www.blueocean.org focuses on sustainability of the oceans first and health risks second.

Web site with fish mercury calculator: www.iatp.org, which has a fish calculator that uses the Environmental Protection Agency's formulas for safe fish consumption for both mercury and PCBs, as well as a person's body weight, amount of fish eaten, and the concentration of contaminants in the fish. The calculator's mercury formula is based on the EPA's estimated "safe" exposure level, or .0001 milligrams per kilogram of body weight per day. For PCBs, the calculator uses the EPA's "safe" exposure level, or 2.0 milligrams per kilogram of body weight per day.

Chapter 5: Environment

Web site about pesticides in foods: http://www.whatsonmyfood.org

Web site with lists of BPA-free cans: http://www.treehugger.com/files/2010/03/7-bpa-free-canned-foods.php; also http://www.ewg.org/reports/bisphenola

Web site about one's personal body burden: http://www.greengoeswitheverything.com/quiz.html

Web site about antibiotics: http://www.keepantibioticsworking.org

Cosmetics

Cosmetic database Web site that can be used to evaluate your shampoo, conditioner, sunscreen and makeup: http://www.ewg.org/skindeep/.

Another useful Web site about cosmetics is http://www.cosmeticsdatabase.com/index

In the Home

Use nontoxic cleaners—good brands include Seventh Generation, Nature Clean, Ecover, Shaklee, Melaleuca, Deidre Imus, Soap Factory AA5 Concentrate, Arm & Hammer Washing Soda, ECOgent

For the environmentally sensitive, use a HEPA filter, especially in your bedroom.

Web site about nontoxic cleaners: http://www.healthylegacy.org/consumereducation

Recipe for Alice's Wonder Spray

2 tablespoons distilled white vinegar

1 teaspoon borax

1½ cups very hot distilled or purified water

¼ cup castile soap or ⅛ cup liquid dish soap

10 to 15 drops essential oils

Directions

Mix the vinegar and borax in a 16-ounce spray bottle.

Fill the bottle with the water and shake to dissolve the vinegar and borax.

Add the soap *last* and then scent with essential oil.

Use as you would any all-purpose cleaner. This mix can get quite soapy, so you might want to have a cloth wet with just water handy to "rinse" with.

Web site about Alice's Wonder Spray: http://www.food.com/recipe/alices-wonder-spray-all-purpose-cleaner-187681#ixzz1lci2OglD

Web site about less toxic household products: http://www.lesstoxicguide.ca/index.asp?fetch=household

Web site about Wonder Spray: http://www.bcbsmnfoundation.org/objects/Tier_3/X17231_Web.pdf

Web site with information about minimizing flame-retardant exposure in mattresses, computers, TVs, carpeting, household furniture, and flooring: http://www.saferproducts.org

Web site about safer chemicals: http://www.saferchemicals.org/toxic-chemicals/flame-retardants.html

Web site with sleep information: http://www.sleepeducation.com

Nontoxic pest control

Web site about nontoxic pest control: http://www.beyondpesticides.org/alternatives/factsheets/index.htm, or hire a professional: http://www.beyondpesticides.org/safetysource/index.htm

General information on environmental health in homes

Web site about healthy houses: http://www.healthybuilding.net

Web site on how to check your local municipal water system: http://www.nytimes.com/toxicwaters

231

Web site on how to filter your water for drinking and cooking: http://www.ewg.org/reports/tapwater/yourwater

Web site on how to seal outdoor wooden structures: http://www.ewg.org/reports/poison-woodsrivers/orderform.php

Web site on how to buy products with natural fibers that are naturally fire-resistant: http://www.ewg.org/reports/pbdefree

Chapter 6: Mind-Body Medicine

Web site with mind-body information: http://www.mind-body-unity.com

Web site with guided imagery CDs on multiple topics including fertility and stress relief: http://www.healthjourneys.com

Web site including "Fertility" CD, stress management, etc.: http://www.tranceformation.com

Chapter 7: Conventional Medicine

Web site of the American Society for Reproductive Medicine: http://www.asrm.org

Web site with further information on fertility issues: http://www.thefertilityadvocate.com

Chapter 9: Ayurveda

Web site to help you determine your own dosha: http://www.banyanbotanicals.com/constitutions

Linda Sparrowe's suggestions for the best poses to enhance fertility:

Yoga (particularly inversions and twists) is believed to balance the endocrine and nervous systems. Some of the most effective poses, according to famed teacher Geeta Iyengar, are Supported Sarvangasana (shoulder stand on a chair); Setu Bandhasana (bridge pose supported with bolsters or blocks); and Sirsasana (headstand), but only if you already have a headstand practice.

The Purpose of Standing Poses

In general, the purpose is to strengthen and tone the whole body and help create balance and stability, and to wake up the body and activate the mind.

On a deeper level, standing poses show us how to stand firm in our own power, to feel strong and capable and confident, and to reach out to the world from the core of our being. They help us to learn how to stand on our own two feet. These poses literally give us a sense of groundedness, which improves the flow of prana (life force) to all channels in the body.

These poses energize the body, open the chest and abdominal area, and extend the spine. They are good for digestive and reproductive health.

Yoga can help correct postural abnormalities and misalignments that often cause symptoms such as headaches, backaches, infertility, and depression. Yoga moves the energy (apana vayu) down and out, which is good for regulating menstruation and reproductive health.

Remember: posture affects thinking, which affects feelings—and vice versa.

The Best Standing Poses for Fertility

Trikonasana (triangle): With its gentle twisting action and grounding properties, this pose increases circulation to the pelvis, and tones and improves functioning of the reproductive and digestive systems.

Parivritta Trikonasana (revolved triangle): With its deeper twist, this pose tones the reproductive organs as well as the kidneys, liver, and spleen; it also increases blood flow to the abdomen and pelvis.

Ardha Chandrasana (half-moon pose): This pose brings healing breath and spaciousness to the abdomen, while allowing it to stay soft and relaxed.

Purpose of Forward Bends

Both standing and seated forward bends soothe and calm the mind and the nervous system including the adrenals, and encourage complete surrender.

On a physical level, forward bends increase flexibility to the hamstrings; take pressure off the lower back (when knees are bent); improve circulation to the legs, pelvis, and kidneys; and release the pelvic-floor muscles.

When done with a concave back, standing forward bends are beneficial for lifting and toning the uterus without gripping or tightening the abdomen.

Supporting the head in forward bends cools down the body and calms the mind. Bending forward helps move the prana through the channels effortlessly and helps regulate agni, the digestive fire in the belly.

Forward bends, like Baddha Konasana (bound angle pose) with head on bolster, allow you to breathe deeply into the belly to help "wake up" the womb, soften the area, and stay with the sensations.

When done with a slight twisting action (not against the belly, but bringing the belly with you), as in Janu Sirsasana (seated head-to-knee pose), forward bends tone and activate the liver, spleen, reproductive organs, and kidneys.

Forward bends help calm anxiety. They bring a sense of safety to the mind and heart, and allow the breath to slow down.

Best Forward Bends for Fertility

Uttanasana (standing forward bend) lifts and tones the uterus, improves circulation to the pelvic area, and relieves agitation and worry.

Prasarita Padottanasana (wide-legged standing forward bend): Practicing with the spine elongated and the head up will lift and tone the uterus and improve circulation to the pelvic area. When releasing the crown of the head down toward floor, the pose will calm jittery nerves.

Janu Sirsasana (seated head-to-knee pose) counteracts the effects of stress on the body and tones and activates reproductive organs, the liver, the spleen, and the kidneys.

Purpose of Backbends

Backbends energize and awaken the front body, stretching the anterior abdominal wall and diaphragm, improving circulation and respiration, and toning and strengthening the back, waist, and side body.

On a deeper level, backbends lift the spirit—they are natural antidepressants—and improve self-confidence. They enhance emotional stability and open the heart to the possibility of conception.

Some backbends tone kidneys and adrenals, which help to regulate menstrual cycle and help prevent water retention.

Backbends can be very powerful. Start with gentle, supported backbends that are soothing and safe (like Supta Baddha Konasana, fully supported, or Setu Bandasana with bolsters, not blocks).

Best Backbends for Fertility

Supta Baddha Konasana (reclining bound angle pose) lifts and tones the uterus, elongates the abdominal area, improves circulation to the pelvic area, and relieves agitation and worry.

Setu Bandha Sarvangasana (bridge pose): This pose is a combination of a backbend and an inversion. If this pose is done on bolsters, it has a soothing effect on the mind and the nervous system. It can be deeply relaxing.

Dhanurasana (bow pose) puts pressure on the abdomen and stretches and elongates the abdomen. Do not do this pose if you think you are already pregnant.

Purpose of Inversions

Going upside down creates balance and stability within your body's systems.

Inversions balance the neuro-endocrine system. In particular, they stimulate blood flow to the brain, activate the pituitary gland and pineal body, and energize the entire physical body. They are very good for jump-starting fertility or getting the menstrual cycle back on track.

Inversions improve posture and lengthen the spine. They also relieve tension in the neck and shoulders.

Some inversions (like Halasana and supported Sarvangasana) can also tame irritability and anxiety.

Inversions can help get us "unstuck" and soothe the nerves. Gentle, supported inversions are best at first—even downward-facing dog, supported shoulder stand (on chair), or supported half plough (Halasana) with legs through a chair.

Best Inversions for Fertility

Viparita Karani: The absolute best pose to do to increase fertility, legs up the wall pose is a deeply relaxing asana. It balances the endocrine system; soothes the nerves; opens up the chest, bringing a sense of calm and joy to the mind and heart; and improves respiration and circulation throughout the body. Some yoga experts believe one should do legs up the wall pose immediately after making love to encourage the semen to stay in the body.

Sarvangasana (shoulder stand): A supported version of shoulder stand is wonderful to alleviate fatigue, nervous energy, and stress. Geeta Iyengar says it helps develop emotional stability, patience, and willpower.

235

Adho Mukha Svanasana (downward-facing dog): All the benefits of inversions for people who don't have a strong inversion practice. Downward-dog gently awakens the whole body, increases circulation, and calms the mind.

Twists

Physically, twists bring flexibility to the spine and hips, and tone and strengthen the abdominals; they also increase mobility in the shoulders and upper back.

Many twists open the chest, which improves circulation and respiration, and decreases depression.

Twists can rejuvenate the liver, kidneys, and spleen, as well as the reproductive organs. They are very beneficial for infertility issues and helping the uterus to return to health after miscarriage.

Avoid all twisting poses during pregnancy—even in the first trimester—with the exception of Bharadvajasana, which can help relieve back pain and increase blood flow to the uterus, adrenals, and ovaries (it is also very beneficial for helping the body heal after miscarriage).

Seated twists can help move emotions that feel stuck. The squeezing and soaking action of a twist moves the stagnant energy out and replaces it with fresh oxygenated blood.

Hip Openers

It is important to open the muscles around the hips and pelvic area.

Try Kapotasana (pigeon pose) on both sides. The pose helps stretch rotator muscles around the hips as well as the hip flexors, and it softens the hips and makes you more flexible.

Do Baddha Konasana (bound angle pose) to open the hips and lift and tone the uterus. This stimulates the reproductive organs as well as the kidneys and bladder, and eases fatigue.

Do Ananda Bakasana (happy baby pose) to calm the mind, gently open the groin, and release the lower back.

Chapter 10: Spirituality

The following are examples of prayers for fertility from various religions.

Christian: St. Gerard's Prayer

Good St. Gerard, powerful intercessor before the throne of God, wonderworker of our day, we call upon you and seek your aid. You know that this marriage has not as yet been blessed with a child, and how much [husband's name] and [wife's name] desire this gift. Please present these fervent pleas to the Creator of life from whom all parenthood proceeds, and beseech Him to bless this couple with a child whom they may raise as His child and heir of heaven. Amen.

(Source: St. Teresita Hospital, Los Angeles, California. Read more at http://www.beliefnet .com/Health/2008/09/Healing-Prayers-for-Infertility.aspx?p=4#ixzz1RstRouTb.)

A prayer from the Judaic tradition:

In You, God, our ancestors trusted,

In You they trusted, and You answered them.

We will trust in God, for God's goodness is never ending; God's mercy is without bounds.

We will trust in God, for God is our help and our shield.

May the God who made heaven and earth, hear our plea and grant us a child.

(Source: "In You, God" poem from RitualWell.org. Based on verses from Song of Songs and Psalm 22. Excerpted from *Lifecycles Volume 1: Jewish Women on Life Passages and Personal Milestones,* ©1998, edited by Debra Orenstein. Read more at http://www.beliefnet.com/ Health/2008/09/Healing-Prayers-for-Infertility.aspx?p=11#ixzz1RSuTa7dg.)

Islamic prayer:

O my Lord! Leave me not childless, though You are the Best of the inheritors,

O my Lord! Grant me from You a good offspring. You are indeed the All-Hearer of invocation.

(Source: *The Noble Quran,* Al-'Imran, 3:38. Read more at http://www.beliefnet.com/ Faiths/Prayer/2009/07/Muslim-Pregnancy-Prayers.aspx?p=3.)

ENDNOTES

Introduction

2 "In 2011, the *New England Journal of Medicine,* reported in the" D. W. Kaufman, J. P. Kelly, L. Rosenberg, T. E. Anderson, and A. A. Mitchell, "Recent Patterns of Medication Use in the Ambulatory Adult Population of the United States: The Slone Survey," *JAMA* 287, no. 3 (January 2002): 337–44.

3 "50 percent of Americans" Lisa A. Croen, Ph.D.; Judith K. Grether, Ph.D.; Cathleen K. Yoshida, M.S.; Roxana Odouli, M.S.P.H.; Victoria Hendrick, M.D., "Antidepressant Use During Pregnancy and Childhood Autism Spectrum Disorders," *Arch General Psychiatry,* July 4, 2011, http://www.ncbi.nlm.nih.gov/pubmed/21727247.

4 "fertility declines and miscarriage rates" B. J. Van Voorhis, "In Vitro Fertilization," *New England Journal of Medicine,* 356 (2007): 379–86.

4 "average age of first" R. Schoen and V. Canudas-Romo, "Timing Effects on First Marriage: Twentieth-Century Experience in England and Wales and the USA," *Popular Studies* 59 (2005): 135–46.

Chapter One: Integrative Medicine Assessment

11 "some research that showed" R. Chang, P. H. Chung, and Z. Rosenwaks, "Role of Acupuncture on the Pregnancy Rate in Patients Who Undergo Assisted Reproduction

Therapy," *Fertility and Sterility* 77, no. 4 (2002): 1149–53; Wolfgang E. Paulus, M.D., Mingmin Zhang, M.D., Erwin Strehler, M.D., et al., "Acupuncture Improves Pregnancy Rate After ART," *Fertility and Sterility* 77, no. 4 (2002): 721–24.

12 "The Eight Principles of Integrative Medicine," http://integrativemedicine.arizona.edu/about/definition.html.

13 "Counterintuitively, a Cochrane review" Z. Alfirevic, D. Devane, and G. M. L. Gyte, "Continuous Cardiotocography (CTG) as a Form of Electronic Fetal Monitoring (EFM) for Fetal Assessment During Labour," *Cochrane Database of Systematic Reviews,* 3 (CD006066) (2006), doi: 10.1002/14651858.CD006066.

14 "On the downside, it increased" H. Gilbert Welch, Lisa Schwartz, and Steven Woloshin, *Overdiagnosed: Making People Sick in the Pursuit of Health* (Boston: Beacon Press, 2012), 105–6.

14 "their immune systems are negatively impacted" J. Neu and J. Rushing, "Cesarean Versus Vaginal Delivery: Long-Term Infant Outcomes and the Hygiene Hypothesis," *Clinics in Perinatology* 38, no. 2 (June 2011): 321–31.

17 "up to 20 percent" M. Freizinger, M. Franko, M. Dacey, et al., "The Prevalence of Eating Disorders in Infertile Women," *Fertility and Sterility* 93, no. 1 (2010): 72–78.

18 "exercise habits" David L. Oliver, "Exercise and Fertility: An Update," *Current Opinion in Obstetrics & Gynecology* 22, no. 4 (2010): 259–63; S. L. Gudmundsdottir, W. D. Flanders, and L. B. Augestad, "Physical Activity and Fertility in Women: The North-Trondelag Health Study," *Human Reproduction* 24, no. 12 (2009): 3196–3204; M. J. De Souza, "Menstrual Disturbances in Athletes: A Focus on Luteal Phase Defects," *Medical Science Sports Exercise* 35, no. 9 (2003): 1553–63.

18 "The ideal BMI for conception" Janet Rich-Edwards, Donna Spiegelman, Miriam Garland, et al., "Physical Activity, Body Mass Index, and Ovulatory Disorder Infertility," *Epidemiology* 13, no. 2 (2003): 184–90.

Chapter Two: Your Body, Your Lifestyle, and Fertility

30 "In response to" Toni Weschler, MPH, *Taking Charge of Your Fertility* (New York: HarperCollins, 2006), 368.

30 "When estrogen blood levels produced" Ibid., 46–48.

31 "When a fertilized egg burrows" Ibid., 50.

34 "For pregnancy to occur" J. B. Stanford, G. L. White, and H. Hatasaka, "Timing Intercourse to Achieve Pregnancy: Current Evidence," *Obstetrics and Gynecology* 100, no. 6 (2002): 1333.

34 "changes in" Victoria Maizes, M.D., and Tieraona Low Dog, M.D., *Integrative Women's Health* (New York: Oxford University Press, 2010), 275–76.

35 "The study found that" T. W. Hilgers, K. D. Daly, A. M. Prebil, and S. K. Hilgers, "Cumulative Pregnancy Rates in Patients with Apparently Normal Fertility and Fertility-Focused Intercourse," *Journal of Reproductive Medicine* 37, no. 10 (October 1992): 864–66.

37 "women who have PCOS" M. T. Sheehan, "Polycystic Ovarian Syndrome: Diagnosis and Management," *Clinical Medicine & Research* 2, no. 1 (2004): 13–27.

37 "Even regularly cycling women" Gretchen S. Davis, Victor Y. Fujimoto, Michael R. Soules, et al., "Reproductive Aging: Accelerated Ovarian Follicular Development Associated with a Monotropic Follicle-Stimulating Hormone Rise in Normal Older Women," *Journal of Clinical Endocrinology and Metabolism* 81, no. 3 (March 1996): 1038–45.

39 "A study that followed" M. J. De Souza, "Menstrual Disturbances in Athletes: A Focus on Luteal Phase Defects," *Medical Science Sports Exercise* 35, no. 9 (2003): 1553–63.

42 "In particular, for every" E. D. Jungheim and K. H. Moley, "Current Knowledge of Obesity's Effects in the Pre- and Periconceptional Periods and Avenues for Future Research," *American Journal of Obstetrics & Gynecology* 203, no. 6 (2010): 525–30.

42 "obesity alters the composition" P. M. Catalano, "Adverse Effects of Obesity on Implantation," *Reproduction* 140, no. 3 (2010): 365–71.

44 "In fact, each hour" Janet W. Rich-Edwards, Donna Spiegelman, Miriam Garland, et al., "Physical Activity, Body Mass Index, and Ovulatory Disorder Infertility," *Epidemiology* 13, no. 2 (2002): 184–90.

44 "reported exercising four hours" S. N. Morris, S. A. Misssmer, D. W. Cramer, et al., "Effects of Lifetime Exercise on the Outcome of In Vitro Fertilization," *Obstetrics and Gynecology* 108, no. 4 (2006): 938–45.

45 "exercise is particularly important" Lauren A. Wise, Kenneth J. Rothman, Ellen M. Mikkelsen, et al., "A Prospective Cohort Study of Physical Activity and Time to Pregnancy," *Fertility and Sterility* 97, no. 5 (May 2012), 1136–41.

45 "Smoking can damage the DNA" Maria Teresa Zenzes, "Smoking and Reproduction: Gene Damage to Human Gametes and Embryos," *Human Reproduction Update* 6, no. 2 (2000): 122–31.

45 "Nicotine can persist in the body" Ibid.

45 "several studies suggest that one year" The Practice Committee of the American Society for Reproductive Medicine, "Smoking and Infertility," *Fertility and Sterility*, 86, supplement, no. 5 (November 2006): S172—S177.

45 "When pregnant women smoke" S. Murin, R. Rafii, and K. Bilello, "Smoking and Smoking Cessation in Pregnancy," *Clinics in Chest Medicine* 32, no. 1 (2011): 75–91.

45 "A meta-analysis showed" C. Augood, "Smoking and Female Infertility: A Systematic Review and Meta-analysis," *Human Reproduction* 13, no. 6 (1998): 1532–39.

46 "If a pregnant woman smokes" G. Penn and L. Owen, "Factors Associated with Continued Smoking During Pregnancy: Analysis of Sociodemographic, Pregnancy and Smoking-Related Factors," *Drug Alcohol Review* 21, no. 1 (2002): 17–25.

46 "one or more drinks a day" Jorge E. Chavarro, M.D., ScD., and Walter C. Willett, M.D., DrPh., *The Fertility Diet* (New York: McGraw-Hill, 2008), 148–49.

46 "Six drinks per day increases" J. C. Sadeu, Claude L. Hughes, Sanjay Agarwal, and Warren G. Foster, "Alcohol, Drugs, Caffeine, Tobacco, and Environmental Contaminant Exposure: Reproductive Health Consequences and Clinical Implications," *Critical Reviews in Toxicology* 40, no. 7 (August 2010): 633–52.

47 "In one study of sixty-eight nurses" S. Labyak, S. Lava, F. Turek, and P. Zee, "Effects of Shiftwork on Sleep and Menstrual Function in Nurses," *Health Care for Women International* 23, nos. 6–7 (2002): 703–14.

47 "In general, we know that" Christina C. Lawson, E. A. Whelan, Hibert Lividoti, et al., "Rotating Shift Work and Menstrual Cycle Characteristics," *Epidemiology* 22, no. 3 (2011): 305–12.

48 "Preliminary research from animal studies" D. F. Kripke, J. A. Elliott , S. D. Youngstedt, et al. "Increased Melatonin and Delayed Offset in Menopausal Depression: Role of Years Past Menopause, Follicle-stimulating Hormone, Sleep End Time, and Body Mass Index," *Journal of Circadian Rhythms* 8, no. 5 (2010), accessed June 10, 2011, http://www.jcircadianrhythms.com/content/5/1/4 doi:10.1186/1740–3391–5–4.

48 "One study exposed" K. V. Danilenko and E. A. Samoilova, "Stimulatory Effect of Morning Bright Light on Reproductive Hormones and Ovulation: Results of a Controlled Crossover Trial," PLOS Clinical Trial 2, no. 2 (2007), doi:10.1371/journal.pctr.0020007.

Chapter Three: Nutrition

58 "low glycemic index" Sandra Woodruff, M.S., R.D., L.D./N, "Glycemic Index," accessed March 7, 2011, http://www.tshc.fus.edu/he/nutrition/Nutrition_Specialneeds.

59 "wonderful set of cookbooks" Jennie Brand-Miller, Thomas M.S. Wolever, Stephen Colagiuri, et al., *The Glucose Revolution* (New York: Da Capo), 1999.

59 "wonderful set" Jennie Brand-Miller, Thomas M.S. Wolever, Stephen Colagiuri, et al., *The Low GI Handbook* (New York: Da Capo), 2004.

59 "wonderful set" Jennie Brand-Miller, Kaye Foster-Powell, Joanna McMillan-Price, *The Low GI Diet Cookbook* (New York: Da Capo), 2005.

60 "Several studies have also shown" "Is Fish Oil a Good Postpartum Depression Treatment?," accessed March 7, 2011, http://www.healthyomega3.com.

60 "women can help prevent" K. P. Su, S. Y. Huang, and T. H. Chiu, "Omega-3 Fatty Acids for Major Depressive Disorder During Pregnancy: Results from a Randomized Double-Blind, Placebo-Controlled Trial," *Journal of Clinical Psychiatry* 69 (2008), 633–34.

61 "These partially hydrogenated" Mayo Clinic Staff, "Transfat Is Double Trouble for Your Heart," accessed March 7, 2011, http://www.mayoclinic.com.

62 "most countries around the world" A. A. Adenie, "Response to Issues on GM Agriculture in Africa: Are Transgenic Crops Safe?," BMC Research Notes 4 (2011), 388; E. W. Wohlers, "Regulating Genetically Modified Food: Policy Trajectories, Political Culture, and Risk Perceptions in the U.S., Canada, and EU," *Politics and the Life Sciences* 29, no. 2 (2010), 17–39.

63 "Overall, the women" Jorge E. Chavarro, M.D., ScD., and Walter C. Willett, M.D., DrPh., *The Fertility Diet* (New York: McGraw-Hill, 2008), 112–13.

64 "in the NHS study" J. E. Chavarro, J. W. Rich-Edwards, B. A. Rosner, and W. C. Willett, "Diet and Lifestyle in the Prevention of Ovulatory Disorder Infertility," *Obstetrics & Gynecology* 110, no. 5 (2007), 1050–58.

64 "The NHS found" J. E. Chavarro, J. W. Rich-Edwards, B. A. Rosner, and W. C. Willett, "Dietary Fatty Acid Intakes and the Risk of Ovulatory Infertility," *American Journal of Clinical Nutrition* 85, no. 1 (2007), 231–37.

65 "Protein had" J. E. Chavarro, J. W. Rich-Edwards, B. A. Rosner, and W. C. Willett, "Protein Intake and Ovulatory Infertility," *American Journal of Obstetrics and Gynecology* 198, no. 2 (2008), 210.

67 "Approximately 3 percent" P. Collin, S. Vilska, P. K. Heinonen, et al., "Infertility and Celiac Disease," *Gut* 39 (1996), 382–84.

67 "The Nurses' Health Study found that carbohydrates" J. E. Chavarro, J. W. Rich-Edwards, B. A. Rossner, and W. C. Willett, "A Prospective Study of Dietary Carbohydrate Quantity and Quality in Relation to Risk of Ovulatory Infertility," *European Journal of Clinical Nutrition* 63 (2009), 78–86.

68 "Cereal companies" David Kessler, *The End of Overeating* (New York: Rodale, 2009), 103.

68 "80 percent of American men" Mehmet Oz, M.D. "Dr. Oz on Nutrional Supplements for Men," accessed March 7, 2011, http://www.oprah.com, June 24, 2009.

69 "Another surprising finding" J. E. Chavarro and Walter C. Willett, M.D., DrPh., *The Fertility Diet,* 109.

70 "If you consume 200 mg" American Academy of Sleep Medicine, "Sleep and Caffeine," accessed March 7, 2011, http://www.sleepeducation.com.

71 "Not All Caffeinated Drinks" http://www.energyfiend.com/the-caffeine-database.

71 "The Nurses' Health Study did point" J. E. Chavarro, J. W. Rich-Edwards, B. A. Rosner, et al., "Caffeinated and Alcoholic Beverage Intake in Relation to Ovulatory Disorder Infertility," *Epidemiology* 20, no. 3 (2009) 374–81.

71 "Data from" Alanna Moshfegh, Joseph Goldman, and Linda Cleveland, "What We Eat in America: Usual Nutrient Intake from Food Compared to Dietary Reference Intakes," Department of Agriculture, Agricultural Resource Service, NHANES (2001–2002).

72 "Avon Longitudinal Study" Joseph R. Hibbeln, M.D. et al, "Maternal Seafood Consumption in Pregnancy and Neurodevelopmental Outcomes in Childhood," *The Lancet* 369, no. 9561 (2007), 578–85.

72 "Another study, of 643 children" Gary J. Myers, Philip W. Davidson, J. J. Strain et al., "Nutrient and Methyl Mercury Exposure from Consuming Fish," *The Journal of Nutrition* 137 (2007), 2805–8.

76 "women convert" G. C. Burdge and S. A. Wootton, "Conversion of Alpha-linolenic Acid to Eicosapentaenoic, Docosapentaenoic and Docosahexaenoic Acids in Young Women," *British Journal of Nutrition* 88, no. 4 (2002):411–420.

76 "Men convert" G. C. Burdge, A. E. Jones, S. A. Wootton, "Eicosapentaenoic and Docosapentaenoic Acids are the Principal Products of Alpha-linolenic Acid Metabolism in Young Men," *British Journal of Nutrition* 88, no. 4 (2002):355–364.

77 "In July 2010" Judy Fahys, "Utah Study Points to Arsenic in Backyard Chickens," *Salt Lake Tribune*, September 21, 2010, accessed March 7, 2011, http://www.saltlaketribune .com.

77 "Fish not only provides" Richard Gray, "Pregnant Women Should Be Allowed to Eat More Fish," *Daily Telegraph,* May 30, 2010, accessed March 7, 2011, http://www.dailytelegraph .com.au.

78 "Raisin exercise" Jon Kabat-Zinn, *Full Catastrophe Living* (New York: Random House, 2006), 27–28. Reprinted with permission.

Chapter Four: Supplements

83 "ROS may also contribute" A. Agarwal , S. Gupta, and R. K. Sharma, "Role of Oxidative Stress in Female Reproduction," *Reproduction Biology Endocrinology* 3, no. 28 (2005): 1–21; M. R. Luck, I. Jeyaseelan, and R. A. Scholes, "Ascorbic Acid and Fertility," *Biology of Reproduction* 52, no. 2 (1995): 262–66.

83 "Women in the study who took multis had a third lower risk of developing ovulatory infertility" J. E. Chavarro, J. W. Rich-Edwards, B. A. Rosner, and W. C. Willett, "Use of Multivitamins, Intake of B Vitamins, and Risk of Ovulatory Infertility," *Fertility and Sterility* 89, no. 3 (March 2008): 668–76.

84 "researchers estimated that 20 percent" A. E. Czeizel, J. Metneki, and I. Dudas, "The Effect of Preconceptional Multivitamin Supplementation on Fertility," *International Journal of Vitamin Nutrition Resources* 66 (1996): 55–58.

84 "Another study found that" P. Lumbiganon, "Multiple-Micronutrient Supplementation for Women During Pregnancy," (Geneva, Switzerland: Reproductive Health Library, World Health Organization, 2007), http://www.who.int/rhl/pregnancy_childbirth/antenatal_care/ nutrition/plcom2/en/index.html (last revised August 23, 2007; accessed April 29, 2009).

84 "multivitamins help prevent birth defects" Y. I. Goh, E. Bollano, T. R. Einarson, and G. Koren, "Prenatal Multivitamin Supplementation and Rates of Congenital Anomalies: A Meta-analysis," *Journal of Obstetrical Gynaecology Canada* 28, no. 8 (2006): 680–89.

84 "taking a multivitamin helps to prevent" Siew S. Lim, Manny Noakes, and Robert J. Norman, "Dietary Effects on Fertility Treatment and Pregnancy Outcomes," *Current Opinion in Endocrinology, Diabetes & Obesity* 14, no. 6 (December 2007): 465–69.

84 "women who take multis during pregnancy " Y. I. Goh and G. Koren, "Prenatal Supple-

mentation with Multivitamins and the Incidence of Pediatric Cancers: Clinical and Methodological Considerations," *Pediatric Blood & Cancer* 50, 2 Supplement (February 2008), doi: 10.1002/pbc.21403.

85 "The CHARGE" Rebecca J. Schmidt, Robin L. Hansen, Jaana Hartiala, et al., "Prenatal Vitamins, One-Carbon Metabolism Gene Variants, and Risk for Autism," *Epidemiology* 22, no. 4 (July 2011): 476–485.

85 "severe language delays" Christine Roth, Per Magnus, Synnve Schjolberg, et al., "Folic Acid Supplements in Pregnancy and Severe Language Delay in Children," *Journal of American Medical Association* 306, no. 14 (October 2011): 1566–73.

88 "evidence that folate" C. Hoyo, A. P. Murtha, J. M. Schildkraut, et al., "Folic Acid Supplementation Before and During Pregnancy in the Newborn Epigenetics Study (NEST)," *BMC Public Health* 11, no. 1 (January 2011): 46.

89 "spells clinical hypothyroidism" B. C. Blount, J. L. Pirkle, J. D. Osterloh, et al., "Urinary Perchlorate and Thyroid Hormone Levels in Adolescent and Adult Men and Women Living in the United States," *Environmental Health Perspectives* 114, no. 12 (2006): 1865–71.

89 "The World Health Organization estimates" Paula M. Gardiner, MD, MPH; Lauren Nelson; Cynthia S. Shellhaas, MD, MPH; et al., "The Clinical Content of Preconception Care: Nutrition and Dietary Supplements," *American Journal of Obstetrics & Gynecology*, Supplement SB 199, no. 6 (December 2008): S345—S356.

89 "If it comes back low" M. B. Zimmermann, P. L. Jooste, and C. S. Pandav, "Iodine Deficiency Disorders," *Lancet* 372, no. 9645 (2008): 1251–62.

89 "to prevent preterm labor" S. Grigoriadis, J. Barrett, R. Pittini, et al., "Omega-3 Supplements in Pregnancy: Are We Too Late to Identify the Possible Benefits?," *Journal of Obstetrics & Gynaecology Canada* 32, no. 3 (March 2010): 209–16.

90 "none were taking the vitamins with omega-3" M. Makrides, "Prostaglandins," *Leukotrienes & Essential Fatty Acids* 81, nos. 2–3 (August_September 2009): 171–74.

90 "In randomized trials" D. Claire Wathes, D. Robert, E. Abayasekara, and R. John Aitken, "Polyunsaturated Fatty Acids in Male and Female Reproduction," *Biology of Reproduction* 77 (2007): 190–201.

90 "In the Nurses' Health Study, women who took iron" J. E. Chavarro, J. W. Rich-Edwards, B. A. Rosner, and W. C. Willetts, "Iron Intake and Risk of Ovulatory Infertility," *Obstetrics & Gynecology* 108, no. 5 (November 2006): 1145–52.

90 "The CDC recommends 18 mg" A. M. Siega-Riz, A. G. Hartzema, C. Turnbull, et al., "The Effects of Prophylactic Iron Given in Prenatal Supplements on Iron Status and Birth Outcomes: A Randomized Controlled Trial," *American Journal of Obstetrics & Gynecology* 194, no. 2 (February 2006): 512–19.

91 "Many women have low vitamin D levels" S. Lewis, R. M. Lucas, J. Halliday, and A. L. Ponsonby, "Vitamin D deficiency and Pregnancy: From Preconception to Birth," *Molecular Nutrition & Food Research* 54, no. 8 (August 2010): 1092–1102.

91 "a recent study showed that lead levels" A. S. Ettinger, "Effect of Calcium Supplementation on Blood Lead Levels in Pregnancy: A Randomized Control Trial," *Environmental Health Perspectives* (2008), doi:10.1289/ehp.11868.

92 "Normally the human digestive tract" J. L. Kaplan, H. N. Shi, and W. A. Walker, "The Role of Microbes in Developmental Immunologic Programming," *Pediatric Research* 69, no. 6 (June 2011): 465–72.

92 "Antioxidants accumulate" M. R. Luck, I. Jeyaseelan, and R. A. Scholes, "Ascorbic Acid and Fertility," *Biology Reproduction* 52 (1995): 262–66.

92 "One study that supports the use of vitamin C" H. Henmi, T. Endo, Y. Kitajima, et al., "Effects of Ascorbic Acid Supplementation on Serum Progesterone Levels in Patients with Luteal Phase Defect," *Fertility and Sterility* 80, no. 2 (2003): 459–61.

93 "Another study, which treated women undergoing IVF" I. Crha, D. Hruba, P. Ventruba, et al., "Ascorbic acid and infertility treatment," *Central European Journal of Public Health* 11 (2003): 63–67.

93 "The pilot study involved" L. M. Westphal, A. S. Trant, and S. B. Mooney, "A Nutritional Supplement for Improving Fertility in Women," *Journal of Reproductive Medicine* 49 (2004): 289–93.

93 "In 2006, the study was" L. M. Westphal, M. L. Polan, and A. S. Trant, "Double-Blind, Placebo-Controlled Study of Fertilityblend: A Nutritional Supplement for Improving Fertility in Women," *Clinical & Experimental Obstetrics & Gynecology* 33, no. 4 (2006): 205–8.

93 "Another antioxidant supplement to" A. Y. Rizk, M. A. Bedaiwy, and H. G. Al-Inany, "N-acetyl-cysteine Is a Novel Adjuvant to Clomiphene Citrate in Clomiphene Citrate-Resistant Patients with Polycystic Ovary Syndrome," *Fertility and Sterility* 83, no. 2 (February 2005): 367–70.

94 "this is another supplement" A. Badawy, O. State, and S. Abdelgawad, "*N*-Acetyl Cyste-

ine and Clomiphene Citrate for Induction of Ovulation in Polycystic Ovary Syndrome: A Cross-over Trial," *Acta Obstetricia et Gynecologica Scandinavica* 86, no. 2 (2007): 218–22.

95 "*Vitex* has been studied" Kimberly Braxton Lloyd, PharmD, and Lori B. Hornsby, PharmD, BCPS, "Complementary and Alternative Medications for Women's Health Issues," *Nutrition in Clinical Practice* 24, no. 5 (October/November 2009): 589–608.

95 "pregnancy rate in ninety-six women" I. I. Gerhard, A. Patek, B. Monga, et al., "Matodynon® for Female Sterility [abstract in English]," *Forsch Komplementarmed* 5 (1998): 272–78.

95 "A smaller trial, of fifty-two women" A. Milewicz, E. Gejdel, H. Sworen, et al., "*Vitex agnus castus* Extract in the Treatment of Luteal Phase Defects Due to Latent Hyperprolactinemia: Results of a Randomized Placebo-Controlled Double-Blind Study [abstract in English]," *Arzneimittelforschung* 43 (1993): 752–56.

99 "A 2010 meta-analysis reviewed" M. G. Showell, J. Brown, A. Yazdani, et al., "Antioxidants for Male Subfertility," *Cochrane Database of Systematic Reviews* 1 (CD007411) (2011), doi: 10.1002/14651858.CD007411.pub2.

99 "When men took antioxidants" S. J. Roseff, "Improvement in Sperm Quality and Function with French Maritime Pine Tree Bark Extract," *Journal of Reproductive Medicine* 47, no. 10 (February 2002): 821–24; A. Schachter, S. Friedman, J. A. Goldman, and B. Ekerman, "Treatment of Oligospermia with the Amino Acid Arginine," *Journal of Urology* 11, no. 5 (1973): 206–9; M. Scibona, P. Meschini, S. Capparelli S, et al., "L-arginine and Male Infertility," *Minerva Urology* 46, no. 4 (1994): 251–53; A. Netter, R. Hartoma, and K. Nahoul, "Effect of Zinc Administration on Plasma Testosterone, Dihydrotestosterone, and Sperm Count," *Archives of Andrology* 7, no. 1 (1981): 69–73; M. Tikkiwal, R. L. Ajmera, and N. K. Mathur, "Effect of Zinc Administration on Seminal Zinc and Fertility of Oligospermic Males," *Indian Journal of Physiological Pharmacology* 31, no. 1 (1987): 30–34; E. B. Dawson, W. A. Harris, W. E. Rankin, et al., "Effect of Ascorbic Acid Supplementation on the Sperm Quality of Smokers," *Fertility and Sterility* 58, no. 5 (1992): 1034–39; E. Kessopoulou, H. J. Powes, K. K. Sharma, et al., "A Double-Blind Randomized Placebo Cross-Over Controlled Trial Using the Antioxidant Vitamin E to Treat Reactive Oxygen Species Associated with Male Infertility," *Fertility and Sterility* 64 (1995): 825–31; A. Lewin and H. Lavon, "The Effect of Coenzyme Q-10 on Sperm Motility and Function," *Molecular Aspects of Medicine* 18, no. 1 (1997): S213—S219;

G. Balercia, F. Mosca, F. Mantero, et al., "Coenzyme Q(10) Supplementation in Infertile Men with Idiopathic Asthenospermia: An Open, Uncontrolled Pilot Study," *Fertility and Sterility* 81, no. 1 (2004): 93–98; W. Y. Wong, H. M. Merkus, C. M. Thomas, et al., "Effects of Folic Acid and Zinc Sulfate on Male Factor Subfertility: A Double-Blind, Randomized, Placebo-Controlled Trial," *Fertility and Sterility* 77, no. 3 (2002): 491–98; A. Agarwal and L. H. Sekhon, "The Role of Antioxidant Therapy in the Treatment of Male Infertility," *Human Fertility* (Cambridge) 13, no. 4 (2010): 217–25.

99 "Men who were treated with a combination" W. Y. Wong, H. M. Merkus, C. M. Thomas, et al., "Effects of Folic Acid and Zinc Sulfate on Male Factor Subfertility: A Double-Blind, Randomized, Placebo-Controlled Trial," *Fertility and Sterility* 77, no. 3 (2002): 491–98.

100 "An antioxidant-supplement study" H. Ghanem, O. Shaeer, and A. El-Segini, "Combination Clomiphene Citrate and Antioxidant Therapy for Idiopathic Male Infertility: A Randomized Controlled Trial," *Fertility and Sterility* 93, no. 7 (May 2010): 2232–35.

100 "One study compared the sperm" M. R. Safarinejad, S. Y. Hosseini, F. Dadkhah, and M. A. Asgari, "Relationship of Omega-3 and Omega-6 Fatty Acids with Semen Characteristics, and Antioxidant Status of Seminal Plasma: A Comparison Between Fertile and Infertile Men," *Clinical Nutrition* 29, no. 1 (February 2010): 100–5.

100 "increased risk of autism" D. K. Kinney, D. H. Barch, B. Chayka, et al., "Environmental Risk Factors for Autism: Do They Help Cause de Novo Genetic Mutations That Contribute to the Disorder?," *Medical Hypotheses* 74, no. 1 (January 2010): 102–6.

Chapter Five: Environment

104 "Several studies have shown" Chensheng Lu, Kathryn Toepel, Rene Irish, et al., "Organic Diets Significantly Lower Children's Dietary Exposure to Organophosphorus Pesticides," *Environmental Health Perspectives* 114, no. 2 (February 2006): 260–63.

104 "Environmental Working Group" Peter Fimrite, "Chemicals, Pollutants Found in Newborns," *San Francisco Chronicle,* December 3, 2009.

107 "EPA has identified seventy-three suspect pesticides" United States Environmental Protection Agency, "Draft List of Initial Pesticide Active Ingredients and Pesticide Inerts to be Considered for Screening under the Federal Food, Drug, and Cosmetic Act," 2007. EPA-HQ-OPPT-2004–0109.

107 "Beyond Pesticides has a list of these chemicals" N. Harriott and J. Feldman, "Pesticides That Disrupt Endocrine System Still Unregulated by EPA," *Pesticides and You* 28, no. 1 (2008): 11–14.

109 "BPA is in many of our plastic" Leon Earl Gray, Jr., "Xenoendocrine Disrupters: Laboratory Studies on Male Reproductive Effects," *Toxicology Letters* 102–103 (December 1998): 331–35.

109 "Plastic wrap can leach" David Wallinga, M.D., and Victoria Maizes, M.D., "Foraging for Healthy Food in the Global Economy: Ten Steps We Can All Take," *Explore: The Journal of Science and Healing* 4, no. 6 (2008): 385–88.

109 "(BPA), an endocrine disruptor" Akingbemi, et al., "Inhibition of Testicular Steroidogenesis by the Xenoestrogen Bisphenol A Is Associated with Reduced Pituitary Luteinizing Hormone Secretion and Decreased Steroidogenic Enzyme Gene Expression in Rat Leydig Cells," *General Endocrinology* 145, no. 2 (February 2004): 592; M. Ema, S. Fujii, M. Furukawa, et al., "Rat Two-Generation Reproductive Toxicity Study of Bisphenol A.," *Reproduction and Toxicology* 15, no. 5 (2001): 505–23; G. M. Gray, J .T. Cohen, G. Cunha, et al., "Weight of the Evidence Evaluation of Low-Dose Reproductive and Developmental Effects of Bisphenol A," *Human Ecology Risk Assessment* 10, no. 5 (2004): 875–921; National Toxicology Program Center for the Evaluation of Risks to Human Production (NTP-CERHR), "NTP-CERHR Panel Report on Reproductive and Developmental Toxicity of Bisphenol A," November 26, 2007, http://cerhr. niehs.nih.gov/ chemicals/bisphenol/BPAFinalEPVF112607.pdf.

109 "(BPA) . . . linked to increased miscarriages" M. Sugiura-Ogasawara, Y. Ozaki, S. Sonta, et al., "Exposure to Bisphenol A Is Associated with Recurrent Miscarriage," *Human Reproduction* 20, no. 23 (2005): 25–29.

109 "similar to diethylstilbestrol (DES)" L. Titus-Ernstoff, R. Troisi, E. E. Hatch, et al., "Menstrual and Reproductive Characteristics of Women Whose Mothers Were Exposed in Utero to Diethylstilbestrol (DES)," *International Journal of Epidemiology* 35 (2006): 862–68; J. Blatt, Le L. Van, T. Weiner, and S. Sailer, "Ovarian Carcinoma in an Adolescent with Transgenerational Exposure to Diethylstilbestrol," *Journal of Pediatric Hematology and Oncology* 25, no. 8 (2003): 635–36.

109 "discovered to cause birth defects" H. Klip, J. Verloop, J.D. van Gool, et al., "Hypospadias in Sons of Women Exposed to Diethylstilbestrol in Utero: A Cohort Study,"

Lancet 359, no. 9312 (2002): 1102–7; M. M. Brouwers, W. F. Feitz, L. A. Roelofs, et al. "Hypospadias: A Transgenerational Effect of Diethylstilbestrol?," *Human Reproduction* 21, no. 3 (2006): 666–69.

109 "Over 90 percent" A. M. Calafat, X. Ye, L. Y. Wong, et al., "Exposure of the U.S. Population to Bisphenol A and 4-*tertiary*-octylphenol, 2003–2004," *Environmental Health Perspectives* 116, no. 1 (January 2008): 39–44.

110 "findings of a 2011 study" K. Ji, et al., "Influence of a Five-Day Vegetarian Diet on Urinary Levels of Antibiotics and Phthalate Metabolites," *Environmental Research* 110, no. 4 (2010): 375–82.

110 "Phthalate urine levels" Tracy J. Woodruff, Ph.D., MPH; Alison Carlson; Jackie M. Schwartz, MPH; and Linda C. Giudice, M.D., Ph.D., "Proceedings of the Summit on Environmental Challenges to Reproductive Health and Fertility," *Fertility and Sterility* 89, no. 1 (February 2008), 281–300.

110 "A 2010 study had similarly" R. A. Rudel, J. M. Gray, C. L. Engel, et al., "Food Packaging and Bisphenol A and Bis(2-Ethyhexyl) Phthalate Exposure: Findings from a Dietary Intervention," *Environmental Health Perspectives* 119, no. 7 (2010): 914–920.

111 "The combination of chlorine" CDC Perchlorate Fact Sheet, http://www.cdc.gov/nceh/publications/factsheets/perchlorate.htm.

111 "can also contain cadmium, lead" S. Telisman, P. Cvitkovic, J. Jurasovic, et al., "Semen Quality and Reproductive Endocrine Function in Relation to Biomarkers of Lead, Cadmium, Zinc, and Copper in Men," *Environmental Health Perspectives* 108, no. 1 (2000): 45–53.

111 "*The New York Times*" Charles Duhigg, "Toxic Waters Clean Water Laws Are Neglected, at a Cost in Suffering," *The New York Times,* September 13, 2009.

113 "Synthetic musks such as" J. Reiner, et al., "Synthetic Musk Fragrances in Human Milk from the United States," *Environmental Science and Technology* 41, no. 11 (2007): 3815–20.

114 "To improve indoor air" R. M. Whyatt, D. B. Barr, D. E. Camann, et al., "Association of *In Utero* Contemporary-Use Pesticides in Personal Air Samples during Pregnancy and Blood Samples at Delivery Among Urban Minority Mothers and Newborns," *Environmental Health Perspectives* 111, no. 5 (2003): 749–56.

114 "The Columbia Center" D. Kass, W. McKelvey, E. Carlton, et al., "Effectiveness of an Integrated Pest Management Intervention in Controlling Cockroaches, Mice and Aller-

gens in New York City Public Housing," *Environmental Health Perspectives* 117, no. 8 (2009): 1219–25.

114 "Maternal exposure to domestic" A. G. Davidson, et al., "Chronic Inhalation Exposure to Cadmium Particulates Was Associated with Changes in Pulmonary Function and Chest Radiographs that Were Consistent with Emphysema," *Lancet* 231, no. 8587 (March 1988): 663–67; Claire Infante-Rivard, Damian Labuda, Maja Krajinovic, and Daniel Sinnett, "Risk of Childhood Leukemia Associated with Exposure to Pesticides and with Gene Polymorphisms," *Epidemiology* 10, no. 5 (September 1999): 481–87; F. I. Sharara, D. B. Seifer, J. A. Flaws, "Environmental Toxicants and Female Reproduction," *Fertility and Sterility* 70, no. 4 (October 1998): 613–22.

114 "lower sperm counts" S. M. Duty et al., "Phthalate Exposure and Human Semen Parameters," *Epidemiology* 14, no. 3 (2003): 269–77; G. Pan et al., "Decreased Serum Free Testosterone in Workers Exposed to High Levels of Di-n-butyl Phthalate (DBP) and Di-2-ethylhexyl Phthalate (DEHP): A Cross-Sectional Study in China," *Environmental Health Perspectives* 114, no. 11 (November 2006): 1643–48; S. Kumar, "Occupational Exposure Associated with Reproductive Dysfunction," *Journal of Occupational Health* 46, no. 1 (2004): 1–19.

114 "men living in agricultural areas" A. Oliva, A. Spira, and L. Multigner, "Contribution of Environmental Factors to the Risk of Male Infertility," *Human Reproduction* 16, no. 8 (2001): 1768–76; S. H. Swan, R. L. Kruse, F. Liu, et al., "Semen Quality in Relation to Biomarkers of Pesticide Exposure," *Environmental Health Perspectives* 111, no. 12 (2003): 1478–84.

115 "In May 2011" Sharon Begley, "Is that a Cellphone in Your Pocket?" *The Daily Beast*, June 2, 2011, http://www.thedailybeast.com/articles/2011/06/02/do-cell-phones-cause-infertility .html.

115 "Cleveland Clinic" Ashok Agarwal, Fnu Deepinder, Rakesh K. Sharma, et al., "Effect of Cell Phone Usage on Semen Analysis in Men Attending Infertility Clinic: An Observational Study," *Fertility and Sterility* 89, no. 1 (2008): 124–28.

116 "30 percent decrease" Kim G. Harley, Amy R. Marks, Jonathan Chevrier, et al., "PBDE Concentrations in Women's Serum and Fecundability," *Environmental Health Perspectives* 118, no. 5 (2010): 699–704.

Chapter Six: Mind-Body Medicine

125 "In addition, when we are stressed" S. Whirledge and J. A. Cidlowski, "Glucocorticoids, Stress, and Fertility," *Minerva Endocrinologica* 35, no. 2 (2010): 109–25.

125 "Dr. Sarah Berga . . ." Sarah L. Berga and T. L. Loucks, "Use of Cognitive Behavior Therapy for Functional Hypothalamic Amenorrhea," *Annals of the New York Academy of Sciences* 1092 (2006): 114–29.

125 "Dr. Berga has shown that . . ." Sarah Berga, "The Diagnosis and Treatment of Stress-Induced Anovulation," *Minerva Ginecology* 57, no. 1 (2005): 45–54.

125 "In contrast . . ." Sarah L. Berga, "Beyond the Obvious: Why Behavioral Interventions Matter," *Menopause* 16, no. 2 (2009): 229–30.

126 "In 2003, she enrolled" W. Tschugguel and Sarah L. Berga, "Treatment of Functional Hypothalamic Amenorrhea with Hypnotherapy," *Fertility and Sterility* 80, no. 4 (October 2003): 982–85; Sarah L. Berga, M. D. Marcus, T. L. Loucks, et al., "Cognitive Behavioral Therapy Can Lead to Full Ovarian Function," *Fertility and Sterility* 80, no. 4 (2003): 976–81.

126 "One surprising finding" Nancy I. Williams, Sarah L. Berga, and Judy L. Cameron, "Synergism Between Psychosocial and Metabolic Stressors: Impact on Reproductive Function in Cynomolgus Monkeys," *American Journal of Physiology, Endocrinology and Metabolism* (00108) (2007), doi: 10.1152/ajpendo.

139 "Research shows that writing about stressful" James W. Pennebaker, Janice K. Kiecolt-Glaser, and Ronald Glaser, "Disclosure of Traumas and Immune Function," *Journal of Consulting and Clinical Psychology* 56, no. 2 (1988): 239–45.

140 "on par with HIV or cancer" A. D. Domar, P. C. Zuttermeister, and R. Friedman, "The Psychological Impact of Infertility: A Comparison with Patients with Other Medical Conditions," *Journal of Psychosomatic Obstetrics & Gynecology* 14 Supplement (1993): 45–52.

140 "One survey looked at" C. J. Nelson, A. W. Shindel, C. K. Naughton, et al., "Prevalence and Predictors of Sexual Problems, Relationship Stress and Depression in Female Partners of Infertile Couples," *Journal of Sexuality and Medicine* 5, no. 8 (2008): 1907–14.

140 "Dr. Alice Domar used a mind-body" Alice D. Domar, D. Clapp, E. A. Slawsby, et al., "Impact of Group Psychological Interventions on Pregnancy Rates in Infertile Women," *Fertility and Sterility* 73, no. 4 (April 2000): 805–11; Alice D. Domar, "Impact of a

Group Mind/Body Intervention on Pregnancy Rates in IVF Patients," *Fertility and Sterility* 95, no. 7 (2011): 2269–73.

140 "They have found that" G. M. D. Lemmens, M. Vervaeke, P. Enzlin, et al., "Coping with Infertility: A Body-Mind Group Intervention Programme for Infertile Couples," *Human Reproduction* 19, no. 8 (2004): 1917–23.

140 "Researcher Dr. Jacky Boivin" Jacky Boivin, "A Review of Psychosocial Interventions in Infertility," *Social Science & Medicine* 57, no. 12 (December 2003): 2325–41.

140 "A second meta-analysis . . ." K. Hammerli, H. Znoj, and J. Barth, "The Efficacy of Psychological Interventions for Infertile Patients: A Meta-analysis Examining Mental Health and Pregnancy Rate," *Human Reproduction* 15, no. 3 (2009): 279–95.

141 "the experience of nineteen Israeli women" Paula Gerber-Epstein, Ronit D. Leightentritt, and Yael Benyamini, "The Experience of Miscarriage in First Pregnancy: The Women's Voices," *Death Studies* 33, no. 1 (2009): 1–29.

142 "In one large study" Lone Schmidt, Bjorn Holstein, Ulla Christensen, and Jacky Boivin, "Does Infertility Cause Marital Benefits?," *Patient Education and Counseling* 59 (PII: S0738–3991(05)00239–9) (2005), doi 10.1016/j.pec.2005.05.015.

Chapter Seven: Conventional Medicine

152 "anti-Mullerian hormone" C. Kunt, G. Ozaksit, Kurt R. Keskin, et al., "Anti-Mullerian Hormone Is a Better Marker than Inhibin B, Follicle Stimulating Hormone, Estradiol, or Antral Follicle Count in Predicting the Outcome of In Vitro Fertilization," *Archives of Gynecology & Obstetrics* 283, no. 6 (June 2011): 1415–21.

155 "The 2010 FASTT Study" R. H. Reindollar, M. M. Regan, P. J. Neumann, et al., "A Randomized Clinical Trial to Evaluate Optimal Treatment for Unexplained Infertility: The Fast Track and Standard Treatment (FASTT) Trial," *Fertility and Sterility* 94, no. 3 (August 2010): 888–99.

155 "increasing the risk of ovarian cancer" F. E. van Leeuwen, H. Klip, T. M. Mooij, et al., "Risk of Borderline and Invasive Ovarian Tumours After Ovarian Stimulation for In Vitro Fertilization in a Large Dutch Cohort," *Human Reproduction* (2011), doi: 10.1093/humrep/der322.

155 "A recent study from Finland" Sari Koivurova, Anna-Liisa Hartikainen, Mika Gissler, et

al., "Neonatal Outcome and Congenital Malformations in Children Born After In-Vitro Fertilization," *Human Reproduction* 17, no. 5 (September 2001), 1391–98.

156 "He points out that in general" The Committee on Gynecologic Practice of the American College of Obstetricians and Gynecologists and the Practice Committee of the American Society for Reproductive Medicine, "Age-Related Fertility Decline—a Committee Opinion," *Fertility and Sterility* 90, no. 3 (2008): 486–87.

Chapter Eight: Traditional Chinese Medicine

162 "An Australian study" M. Coyle and C. Smith, "Survey Comparing TCM Diagnosis, Health Status and Medical Diagnosis in Women Undergoing Assisted Reproduction," *Acupuncture in Medicine* 23, no. 2 (2005): 62–69.

172 "There are three postulated" W. Paulus, M. Zhang, E. Strehler, et al., "Influence of Acupuncture on the Pregnancy Rate in Patients Who Undergo Assisted Reproductive Therapy," *Fertility and Sterility* 77, no. 4 (2002): 721–24.

172 "A meta-analysis, or review" Eric Manheimer, Grant Zhang, Laurence Udoff, et al., "Effects of Acupuncture on Rates of Pregnancy and Live Birth Among Women Undergoing In Vitro Fertilisation: Systematic Review and Meta-analysis," *British Medical Journal* 336, no. 535 (2008): 1–8.

173 "the protocol of Dr. Wolfgang Paulus" Wolfgang E. Paulus, M.D., Mingmin Zhang, M.D., Erwin Strehler, M.D., et al., "Influence of Acupuncture on the Pregnancy Rate in Patients Who Undergo Assisted Reproduction Therapy," *Fertility and Sterility* 77, no. 4 (April 2002): 721–24.

173 "Dr. Magarelli did a retrospective" Paul C. Magarelli, M.D., Diane K. Cridennda, and Mel Cohen, "Changes in Serum Cortisol and Prolactin Associated with Acupuncture During Controlled Ovarian Hyperstimulation in Women Undergoing In Vitro Fertilization—Embryo Transfer Treatment," *Fertility and Sterility* 92, no. 6 (2009): 1870–79.

173 "In a small study" S. DeLacey, C. Smith, and C. Paterson, "Building Resilience: A Preliminary Exploration of Women's Perceptions of the Use of Acupuncture as an Adjunct to In Vitro Fertilisation," *BMC Complementary & Alternative Medicine* 9, no. 50 (2009): 54.

177 "Small studies show" J. A. Stone, K. K. Yoder, and E. A. Case, "Delivery of a Full-Term Pregnancy After TCM Treatment in a Previously Infertile Patient Diagnosed with Poly-

cystic Ovary Syndrome," *Alternative Therapies in Health & Medicine* 15, no. 1 (2009): 50–52; H. Sang, "Clinical and Experimental Research into Treatment of Hysteromyoma with Promoting Qi Flow and Blood Circulation, Softening and Resolving Hard Lump," *Traditional Chinese Medicine* 24, no. 4 (2004): 274–79; Fritz Wieser, Misha Cohen, Andrew Gaeddert, et al., "Evolution of Medical Treatment for Endometriosis: Back to the Roots?" *Human Reproduction Update* 13, no. 5 (2007): 487–99.

177 "One encouraging study" Shi Jian-jun et al., "Clinical Observations on a Four-Step Method for Regulating Menstruation on Improving the Adverse Effects After Clomiphene Induction of Ovulation," *Zhe Jiang Zhong Yi Za Zhi (Zhejiang Journal of Chinese Medicine)* 7, no. 405 (2007): 73.

Chapter Nine: Ayurveda

181 "Vata is necessary" Premal Patel, M.D., "Ayurveda," in *Integrative Women's Health,* ed. Victoria Maizes, M.D. and Tieraona Low Dog, M.D. (New York: Oxford University Press, 2010), 111–16.

186 "One study found that" S. A. Dayani Siriwardene, L. Karunathilaka, N. D. Kodituwakku, and Y. Karunarathne, "Clinical Efficacy of Ayurveda Treatment Regimen on Subfertility with Poly Cystic Ovarian Syndrome (PCOS)," *AYU* 31, no. 1 (2010): 24–27.

187 "Researchers at the Interdisciplinary" M. Gautam, S. Saha, S. Bani, et al., "Immunomodulatory Activity of Asparagus Racemosus on Systemic Th1/Th2 Immunity: Implications for Immunoadjuvant Potential," *J: Journal of Ethnopharmacology* 121, no. 2 (January 2009): 241–47.

188 "In a three-month controlled" Abbas Ali Mahdi, Kamla Kant Shukla, Mohammad Kaleem Ahmad, et al., "Withania Somnifera Improves Semen Quality in Stress-Related Male Fertility," *Evidence-Based Complementary Alternative Medicine* (ID 576962) (July 2009), doi:10.1093/ecam/nep.

188 "A study was done" Kamla Kant Shukla, Abbas Ali Mahdi, Mohammad Kaleem Ahmad, et al., "Mucuna Pruriens Improves Male Fertility by Its Action on the Hypothalamus-Pituitary-Gonadal Axis," *Fertility and Sterility* 92, no. 6 (December 2009): 1934–40.

Chapter Ten: Spirituality

201 "Dr. Rachel Naomi Remen" Rachel Naomi Remen, M.D., "On Defining Spirit," *Noetic Sciences* Review 47, no. 64 (Winter 1998).

215 "religious leaders" Robab Roudsari, "Looking at Infertility Through the Lens of Spirituality," *Human Fertility* 10, no. 3 (September 2007): 141–47.

217 "Praying" from *Thirst* by Mary Oliver, published by Beacon Press, Boston, Massachusetts. Copyright © 2004 by Mary Oliver, used herewith by permission of the Charlotte Sheedy Literary Agency, Inc.

Conclusion

222 "In 2010, a study revealed" Marijana Vujkovic, B.Sc.; Jeanne H. de Vries, Ph.D.; Jan Lindemans, Ph.D., et al., "The Preconception Mediterranean Dietary Pattern in Couples Undergoing In Vitro Fertilization/Intracytoplasmic Sperm Injection Treatment Increases the Chance of Pregnancy," *Fertility and Sterility* 94 (2010): 2096–101.

222 "Alice Domar's 2011 study" Alice D. Domar, "Impact of a Group Mind/Body Intervention on Pregnancy Rates in IVF Patients," *Fertility and Sterility* 95, no. 7 (2011): 2269–70.

223 "the effect they have on future generations" Philippe Grandjean, David Bellinger, Åke Bergman, et al., "The Faroes Statement: Human Health Effects of Developmental Exposure to Chemicals in Our Environment," *Basic & Clinical Pharmacology & Toxicology* 102, no. 2 (2007): 73–75.

223 "Epigenetics reveals" National Research Council, *Scientific Frontiers in Developmental Toxicology and Risk Assessment* (Washington, DC: National Academy Press, 2000).

BIBLIOGRAPHY

Adrienne, Helen. *On Fertile Ground: Healing Infertility*. New York: CreateSpace, 2010.

Benson, Herbert. *The Relaxation Response*. New York: HarperCollins, 2000.

Brand Miller, Jennie, Thomas M.S. Wolever, Stephen Colagiuri, and Janette Brand Miller. *The Glucose Revolution*. New York: Marlowe & Company, 2006.

Brand Miller et al. *The Low GI Handbook*. New York: Da Capo, 2004.

Brand Miller et al. *The Low GI Diet Cookbook*. New York: Da Capo, 2005.

Chavarro, MD, ScD, E. Jorge, and Walter C. Willett, MD, DrPh, *The Fertility Diet*. New York: McGraw-Hill, 2008.

Domar, Alice. *Healing Mind, Healthy Woman*. New York: Penguin, 1997.

Domar, Alice. *Conquering Infertility*. New York: Penguin, 2004.

Indichova, Julia. *Inconceivable: A Woman's Triumph over Despair and Statistics*. New York: Three Rivers Press, 2001.

Kabat-Zinn, Jon. *Coming to Our Senses*. New York: Hyperion, 2006.

Kessler, David. *The End of Overeating*. New York: McClelland & Stewart, 2009.

Lewis, Randine A. *The Infertility Cure: The Ancient Chinese Wellness Program for Getting Pregnant and Having Healthy Babies*. New York: Little, Brown, 2005.

Maizes, Victoria M.D. and Tieraona Low Dog, M.D., *Integrative Women's Health*. New York: Oxford University Press, 2010.

Mundy, Liza. *Everything Conceivable: How the Science of Assisted Reproduction Is Changing Our World.* New York: Knopf, 2008.

Pollan, Michael. *In Defense of Food.* New York: Penguin, 2009.

Pollan, Michael. *Food Rules.* New York: Penguin, 2009.

Nhat Hahn, Thich. *The Miracle of Mindfulness.* New York: Beacon, 1999.

Singer, Pete and Jim Mason. *The Ethics of What We Eat: Why Our Food Choices Matter.* New York: Rodale, 2007.

Sparrowe, Linda. *The Woman's Book of Yoga and Health.* New York: Shambhala, 2002.

Weschler, Toni. *Taking Charge of Your Fertility, 10th Anniversary Edition.* New York: Collins, 2006.

Weil, Andrew, and Rosie Daley. *The Healthy Kitchen: Recipes for a Better Body, Life, and Spirit.* New York: Knopf, 2002.

INDEX

abortions, 17, 22, 95
acanthosis Nigricans, 39
Accutane, 18, 149
activism, 223
acupuncture
    fear of, 14
    integrative medicine and, 3,
        13, 14
    IVF and, 156, 158, 172–74
    men and, 177
    menstrual cycle and, 171–72
    mind-body connection and,
        122, 223
    miscarriages and, 176
    number of treatments of, 171
    relaxation and, 172, 173
    reproductive physiology and, 28
    secondary infertility story
        and, 11
    spirituality and, 216, 217
    stress and, 172, 173
    TCM and, 161, 169, 171–76,
        177
    treatment selections and, 24
    West fertility journey and,
        194–96
    yin and yang and, 172

adoption, 211, 218, 222
adrenal glands, 28, 124, 125,
    126, 188
Adrienne, Helen, 127, 136, 139,
    141–42, 143, 144
age
    difficulty with conception
        and, 151
    freezing eggs and, 158
    FSH and, 37–38
    and ideal age to have a baby,
        3–4
    influence on pregnancy of,
        38–39
    IVF and, 156, 157
    ovulation predictor kits and,
        37
    principles of integrative
        medicine and, 222
    reproductive physiology and,
        35, 37–38
    reproductive technologies and,
        223
    TCM and, 163–64, 165, 166,
        167
agni (digestion), 183, 185,
    199

Agriculture Department, U.S.,
    59, 186
air pollution, 113–14
alcohol, 21, 46–47, 49, 54, 63,
    77–78, 148, 151, 156
Alice's Wonder Spray, 113
alpha-linolenic acid (ALA), 76,
    89
alternative medicine, 9–10, 12,
    13, 14, 222. *See also specific*
    therapy
Amanda (patient), 51
amenorrhea, 43, 126, 139
American Academy of Family
    Medicine, 88
American Academy of Pediatrics,
    88
American College of
    Obstetricians and
    Gynecologists, 88
American Herbalist Guild, 94
American Society for
    Reproductive Medicine,
    157, 158
AMH (anti-Mullerian hormone),
    152, 156
amniocentesis, 203

INDEX

anatomy: fertility problems and, 40

androgens, 41, 42, 69, 104, 153

anemia, 18, 90, 149, 157

animal husbandry, 65

anti-inflammatories, 39, 99

anti-inflammatory (Mediterranean) diet, 52–63, 68, 222

antibiotics, 65, 92, 110, 149, 154

antidepressant medication (SSRI) study, 2–3

antihistamines, 17, 18

antioxidants, 10, 11, 68–69, 92–93, 99, 100, 148, 151, 188. *See also specific antioxidant*

Anusara, 189, 216

anxiety, 46, 135, 137, 138, 141, 148, 165, 173, 189–90, 192, 216

Arizona Center for Integrative Medicine, 4, 94, 130, 162, 168, 207

aromatherapy, 49

arsenic, 76–77, 105, 111

Artemesia vulgaris (herb), 170

artichoke leaf, 99

artificial insemination, 154–55, 215

Ashoka (herb), 188

ashwaganda (herb), 97, 180, 186, 188

assessment
   of fats in diet, 59–60
   initial physician, 15–20
   personal/self-, 15–16, 20–23, 59–60
   TCM, 223
   of vitamin D, 77

assisted reproduction, 1, 42–43, 215. *See also specific method*

astrology, 180, 216

athletes, 39–40, 43, 44–45

Augustine, Mary Beth, 66–67, 68

autism, 2, 3, 85, 100, 108, 223

Avon Longitudinal Study of Parents and Children, 72

Ayurveda
   agni (digestion) and, 183, 185, 199
   balance (*prakruti*) and, 180–81, 183–85, 186, 187, 190, 197, 198, 199, 200
   basic views of, 180–81
   body and, 179, 180–81, 184, 190, 191, 200
   challenges to pregnancy and, 2
   detoxification and, 180, 198–99
   diet/nutrition and, 180–81, 183, 184, 185, 186–87, 195, 198, 199, 200
   dinacharya (wisdom of daily routine) of, 184
   doshas of, 180–83, 184, 185, 186, 189, 198, 200
   fertility and, 185–89
   herbs and, 95, 97, 180, 184, 186, 198–99, 200
   history of, 180, 200
   importance of, 200
   karma and, 199–200
   marital relationships and, 179, 180, 185
   meditation and, 184, 185, 189–96, 199
   men and, 188, 189, 194
   menstruation/menstrual cycle and, 181, 186, 187, 188, 191, 193, 194
   mind and, 179, 180, 200
   mind-body connection and, 180–81, 185, 189, 193, 194, 197
   moral/ethical practices (*yamas*) of, 184–85
   principles of integrative medicine and, 3, 9, 13
   qi and, 180
   spirit and, 179, 180–81, 200
   stress and, 184, 185, 186, 188
   West fertility journey and, 194–96

Western medicine compared with, 180, 181
   yin and yang and, 180
   yoga and, 180, 184–85, 189–96, 197–98, 199

Ayurvedic Academy (Seattle, Washington), 185

Ayurvedic Institute (Albuquerque, New Mexico), 180, 185

azoospermia, 41

balance
   Ayurveda and, 180–81, 183–85, 186, 187, 190, 197, 198, 199, 200
   TCM and, 161–62, 171–76, 178

Basal Body Temperature (BBT), 23, 30, 31, 32–33, 34, 36, 40, 49, 125, 152

belief system, 19, 136, 137–38, 205. *See also* spirit/spirituality

Benson, Herbert, 128, 133

Berga, Sarah, 125–26, 139

Bergstrom, Roy, 11

beverages, 54, 63, 70–71. *See also type of beverage*

Bhattacharya, Bhaswati, 189, 199

Billings Ovulation Method, 35

birth
   as female initiation, 205
   multiple, 155, 157
   mystery of, 205, 222

birth control, 2, 4, 17, 20, 23–24, 27, 28, 35, 39, 152

birth defects, 21, 46, 84, 85, 87, 92, 109, 114, 155–56, 157

birth rate, U.S., 1

bisphenol A (BPA), 104, 105, 109–10, 111, 149

blame: mind-body connection and, 142–45

blood: TCM and, 163, 165–67, 176

blood pressure, 133, 148, 149, 157
blood sugar, 58, 59, 120, 153, 186, 189
blood tests, 149, 152
body
  Ayurveda and, 179, 180–81, 184, 190, 191, 200
  befriending the, 191
  challenges to pregnancy and, 2
  cleansing and preparing, 179
  conventional medicine and, 8
  definition of integrative medicine and, 7
  importance of being acquainted with, 23–24
  integrative medicine and, 2, 8, 222
  natural healing ability of, 8, 13, 120
  purity of, 184
  self-assessment of, 222
  smiling at your, 131
  yoga and, 191
  See also mind-body connection
Body Mass Index (BMI), 18–19, 22, 42, 63–64
body scanning, 127, 129, 132
Boivin, Jacky, 140
botanicals, 10
brain
  Ayurveda and, 191
  environmental impact on, 104, 107, 108, 115
  fetal, 11, 72, 77–78, 104, 107, 108, 115
  fish oil and, 11
  lifestyle impact on, 46, 48
  mind-body connection and, 124, 125, 139, 143
  nutrition and, 72, 77–78
  supplements and, 89
breast cancer, 76, 104, 109
Breast Cancer Research Foundation, 109–10
breath work
  body scanning and, 132

diaphragmatic, 129–30
  meditation and, 131
  mind-body connection and, 119–20, 127–33, 144, 145
  secondary infertility story and, 11
  sleep and, 49
  TCM and, 168
  yoga/Ayurveda and, 181, 189, 190, 191, 192, 194, 196, 197–98
Brown, Louise, 155
Bupleurum (herb), 99
burdock, 99

cadmium, 111, 112
caffeine, 10, 47, 49, 70, 71
calcium, 86, 87, 91, 96, 149
cancer
  difficulty with conception and, 151
  environmental impact on, 104, 109, 113
  freezing eggs and, 159
  inflammation and, 60
  insulin and, 58
  IVF and, 155
  lifestyle and, 47
  nutrition and, 52, 58, 60, 61, 62, 76
  supplements and, 84, 91
  See also type of cancer
cans as packaging, 109–10
carbohydrates
  high-glycemic-load, 28, 54, 58, 59, 68, 70
  limited, 39
  low-glycemic-load, 53, 58
  nutrition and, 53, 54, 58–59, 64, 65, 67–68, 70
cardiovascular issues, 44, 47, 62, 84
carom seeds, 188
celiac disease, 17, 19, 21, 67, 68, 153
celibacy, 179
cell phones, 115–16

Center for Nutrition Policy, USDA, 59
Centers for Disease Control (CDC), 81, 90, 156
ceremonies/rituals, 3, 13, 179, 188, 205–12, 219, 223
cervical mucus
  acupuncture and, 172
  age and, 35
  changes in, 34, 37
  difficulty with conception and, 152
  identification of most fertile time and, 34
  importance of being acquainted with, 23
  initial assessment and, 17
  mind-body connection and, 125
  nutrition and, 67
  reproductive physiology and, 34, 35, 37
  TCM and, 162, 164, 172, 175, 177
cervix, 30, 34, 35–36. See also cervical mucus
cesarean sections, 14
chakras, 210
chanting, 191, 195, 204
CHARGE (Childhood Autism Risks from Genetics and Environment), 85
chasteberry, 93, 95, 97
chemotherapy, 19, 22, 151, 159, 162
Chiasson, Ann Marie, 207, 209–10
children
  as birthright and blessing, 221
  connection among all women having, 209
  environmental effects on, 104, 106–7
  reasons for wanting to have, 19
chlamydia, 40, 154
cholesterol, 39, 61, 76
chromium, 97

cinnamon, 97
circadian rhythms, 48
Clean Fifteen fruits and
	vegetables, 62, 107
cleaning products, 113
Clearblue Fertility Monitor, 37
Cleveland Clinic, 115
Clomid, 11, 93–94, 100, 121,
	122, 135, 136, 148,
	154–55, 156, 177, 215–16
coffee, 13, 21, 54, 63, 70–71
cognitive behavioral therapy,
	125–26, 134, 140–41
cognitive restructuring, 127,
	134–38
Columbia Center for Children's
	Environmental Health, 114
conception
	conventional medicine and,
		149–50, 151–54
	difficulties with, 151–54
	as mystery, 220
	partners in, 220
	physician discussions about
		likelihood of, 149–50
	potential warnings about
		difficulty of, 150
	as primal urge, 1
	spirituality and, 205, 220
	See also birth
congenital defects, 43, 46
contraception, 17, 20, 28, 91.
	See also birth control
conventional medicine
	basic laboratory work and,
		149–50
	difficulty with conception
		and, 151–54
	freezing eggs and, 158–59
	infertility and, 154–56
	IVF and, 151, 152, 155–58
	likelihood of conception
		discussions and, 149–50
	medications and, 149
	men and, 148, 149, 151, 153,
		154
	mind-body connection and,
		148

preparation for conception
	and, 147–50, 222
principles of IM and, 12, 13,
	14
self-assessment test and,
	21–22
supplements and, 149
as tool for IM physicians, 9
cooking utensils, 110
coping strategies, 142, 202, 214.
	See also personal practice/
	coping strategies
CoQ10, 100
corpus luteum, 30, 31, 39–40,
	125, 153
cortisol, 44, 124, 125, 173, 188
Coryell, Devorah, 136–37
cosmetics, 22, 24, 98, 104, 105,
	112
Coughlin, Kevin, 92
cramps, 34. See also
	mittelschmerz
Creighton Model Fertility Care
	System, 35
critical windows of susceptibility
	concept, 105–6
cumin, 187, 188, 189

dairy products, 64, 69–70,
	170, 171. See also specific
	product
Daley, Nathan, 111, 113
Damiana (Turnera aphrodisiaca),
	95–96
Dan Tian area, 170, 179, 210
dandelion, 99
dental health, 148
depression, 46, 47, 48, 52, 60,
	71, 89, 90, 120, 140, 150,
	166
detoxification, 98–99, 105, 107,
	175, 180, 198–99
DHA (docosahexaenoic acid),
	76, 85–86, 89, 90
diabetes
	conventional medicine and,
		148, 155, 157
	environment and, 104, 109

gestational, 18, 91, 148, 157
initial assessment and, 18
insulin and, 58
IVF and, 155, 157
lifestyle and, 43, 47
maternal, 155
nutrition and, 52, 58, 70
supplements and, 91
diet
	Ayurveda and, 180–81, 183,
		184, 185, 186–87, 195,
		198, 199, 200
	becoming an activist and, 223
	challenges to fertility and, 2
	chemicals in, 19
	detoxification and, 98–99
	fertility problems and, 28, 39,
		40, 49
	gluten-free, 67, 68
	initial assessment and, 17–18
	IVF and, 158, 222
	lifestyle and, 28, 49, 51–52
	mind-body connection and,
		122
	miscarriages and, 186–87
	principles of integrative
		medicine and, 2, 12–13,
		15, 222
	secondary infertility and, 10
	self-assessment test and, 20
	TCM and, 161, 166, 167,
		170–71, 179
	treatment options and, 24
	weight and, 52
	West fertility journey and, 195
	See also anti-inflammatory
		(Mediterranean) diet; food;
		nutrition
Dietary Guidelines for
	Americans (USDA), 59
Dietary Supplement Health and
	Education Act (DSHEA),
	82
Dinacharya Institute (New York
	City), 189
dinacharya (wisdom of daily
	routine), 184
Dirty Dozen, 62, 107

DNA, 45, 88, 92, 113, 223
Domar, Alice, 127, 128, 134, 135, 140, 143, 222
Dong quai (herb), 97
doshas, 180–83, 184, 185, 186, 189, 198, 200. *See also* Kapha; Pitta; Vata
dysmenorrhea, 166, 169, 177

eating disorder case, 135
ectopic pregnancy, 45
Edwards, Robert, 155
egg(s)
    aging of, 38
    donation of, 13
    fertility problems and, 39, 42–43, 45, 152
    freezing, 23, 24, 158–59, 215
    infertility and, 155
    lifestyle impact on, 42–43, 45
    mind-body connection and, 124, 125
    number of, 45
    omega-3 and, 76–77
    organic, 76–77
    principles of integrative medicine and, 13
    quality of, 152
    reproductive physiology and, 30, 31, 34, 35, 38
embryos
    freezing of, 23, 24, 158–59, 215
    IVF and, 156–57
    reproductive physiology and, 31
    treatment options and, 23, 24
EMF (electromagnetic field) exposure, 115–16
emotions
    Ayurveda and, 183, 190, 198
    emotional readiness and, 19
    initial assessment and, 19
    spirituality and, 203, 206
    See also specific emotion
endocrine system, 104, 108, 109, 113, 124, 149

endometriosis, 38, 40, 68, 154, 169, 177, 197–98
endometrium, 30, 31, 39, 40, 172
energy
    Ayurveda and, 179
    herbs and, 97
    spirituality and, 210
    TCM and, 162, 165, 166–67, 168, 169, 170, 171, 174, 176, 177
    yoga and, 191, 192
    See also doshas
energy medicine, 9, 13
environment
    air pollution and, 113–14
    Ayurveda and, 198
    challenges to fertility and, 2
    chemicals and, 106–16
    cleaning products and, 113
    conventional medicine and, 149, 151
    critical windows of susceptibility concept and, 105–6
    detoxification and, 98
    difficulty with conception and, 151
    EMF exposures and, 115–16
    food and, 62, 65, 77, 104, 107–9, 110, 149
    growing awareness about, 98
    inflammation and, 52
    initial assessment and, 19
    lifestyle changes and, 51
    male fertility problems and, 41, 99
    mind-body connection and, 137, 143
    organic foods and, 62
    packaging and, 109–10
    personal care products and, 105, 112–13, 149
    pesticides/insecticides and, 107, 110, 114–15
    precautionary principle concerning, 103–4

principles of integrative medicine and, 2, 15
    reasons for concerns about, 2, 104–5, 222, 223
    regulation of, 103, 110–11
    self-assessment test and, 22
    supplements and, 91
    testing for toxins and, 117
    treatment options and, 24
Environmental Health Perspectives, 110
Environmental Protection Agency (EPA), 71, 72, 73, 103, 104, 107, 110, 111
Environmental Working Group, 104, 107, 112
EPA (eicosopentaenoic acid), 76, 86, 89, 90
epigenetics, 2, 223
erectile dysfunction, 42, 47, 100–101
erythromycin, 149
essence
    definition of, 163
    TCM and, 163–64, 165–67, 170, 171, 176
essential fatty acids, 53, 100. *See also* omega-3 fatty acids
estradiol, 40, 47, 95, 152–53
estrogen
    acupuncture and, 172
    age and, 37
    Ayurveda and, 187
    cervical mucus and, 35
    environmental impact on, 104, 109
    fertility problems and, 39, 41, 42, 44, 99
    herbs and, 95, 187
    lifestyle and, 42, 44
    male fertility problems and, 41, 99
    medications for blocking, 172
    mind-body connection and, 124, 126
    nutrition and, 59, 62, 69
    ovulation predictor kits and, 37

estrogen (*cont.*)
    reproductive physiology and, 30, 35, 37
    synthetic, 109
estrogen mimics, 41
estrone-3-flucutronide, 37
exercise/physical activity
    Ayurveda and, 183, 184
    conventional medicine and, 148, 150
    definition of integrative medicine and, 8
    epigenetics and, 223
    fertility problems and, 28, 39, 40, 43–45, 49
    frequency of, 44
    initial assessment and, 18–19
    intense/extreme, 23, 24, 43, 44, 45, 49
    lifestyle changes and, 51
    men and, 45
    mind-body connection and, 120, 122, 134, 138
    principles of integrative medicine and, 15
    self-assessment test and, 22, 23
    sleep and, 49
    TCM and, 166
    as tool for physicians, 9
    treatment options and, 24

fallopian tubes, 30, 152, 154
family history, 19
fast foods, 2, 54
FASTT Study, 155
fats
    animal, 108–9
    basic nutritional needs of average woman and, 53
    environment and, 108–9
    monounsaturated, 59, 60, 64
    nutrition and, 53, 54, 59–61, 63–64
    polyunsaturated, 59, 60–61, 64
    saturated, 59–60, 61, 69

fears
    Ayurveda and, 190, 191, 192
    initial assessment and, 19
    mind-body connection and, 137–38, 143
    self-assessment test and, 23
    TCM and, 165, 167, 168
fenugreek, 186, 189
fertility
    challenges to, 1–2
    common problems with, 38–41
    peak, 3
    reproductive physiology and, 28–38, 49
    TCM as enhancing, 177–78, 210
    See also specific topic
Fertility Blend, 93, 95
fetal alcohol syndrome, 46
fetal origins research, 104
fetal programming hypothesis, 92
fetus
    environmental impact on, 104, 106–7, 108
    heart monitoring of, 13–14
    lifestyle impacts on, 45–46
fiber, 53, 54, 61, 63, 76, 98
fibroids, 17, 22, 38, 40, 197–98
fish. *See* seafood
fish oil, 11, 86, 90. *See also* omega-3 fatty acids
folic acid
    conventional medicine and, 148, 149, 153
    difficulty with conception and, 153
    initial assessment and, 18
    nutrition and, 88
    self-assessment test and, 21
    as supplement, 82, 84, 85, 86, 88, 99–100, 101
    treatment options and, 24
follicle scans, 154
follicle-stimulating hormones. *See* FSH
follicular phase, 30, 31, 38, 40, 93, 176–77, 186, 193

food
    arsenic in, 76–77
    Ayurveda and, 186, 198
    cold, 170–71, 179
    "dampening," 171
    detoxification and, 98
    environment and, 104, 107–9, 110, 149
    labels on, 65–66, 68, 82–83
    liver-supported, 99
    packaging of, 109–10
    pesticides and, 62
    processed and refined, 110
    TCM and, 170–71, 179
    vitamin D fortified, 77
    See also diet; nutrition; *specific food*
Food and Drug Administration (FDA), U.S., 65, 71, 72, 73, 82, 108, 111, 112
4-7-8 Breath, 130–31, 144
fragrances, 112–13
freezing eggs/embryos, 23, 24, 158–59, 215
Friend, John, 216, 217
fruits and vegetables, 21, 22, 53, 54, 61–62, 68, 107, 186
FSH (follicle-stimulating hormone)
    age and, 37–38
    Ayurveda and, 188
    conventional medicine and, 152, 153, 154, 155, 156, 158
    fertility problems and, 39, 40, 41, 44, 48, 152, 153
    freezing eggs and, 158
    herbs and, 95
    infertility and, 154, 155, 156
    lifestyle and, 44, 48
    male fertility and, 41
    mind-body connection and, 124, 125
    nutrition and, 66
    reproductive physiology and, 30, 37–38
    TCM and, 164

functional hypothalamic amenorrhea, 126, 139

gardening metaphor, 161–62, 193, 210, 219, 220
Garrison, Julianne, 10–12
genetically modified organisms (GMOs), 62–63
genetics, 38, 41, 223
ginseng, 100–101, 180, 188
glucose, 42, 59, 153
gluten-free diet, 67, 68
glutocorticosteroids. *See* cortisol
glycemic index (GI), 58–59
goddesses, fertility, 219–20
gonadotropin-releasing hormones (GnRH), 30, 44, 124, 125, 172
gonorrhea, 153–54
gratitude: developing a sense of, 218
guduchi (herb), 189

hair, 19, 22, 38, 39, 105, 150, 153
Hammerschlag, Carl, 207
Hanh, Thich Nhat, 131
Hannah (biblical woman), 212–13
happiness, 144, 183
harmony. *See* balance
HCG (human chorionic gonadotropin), 11, 31, 42–43, 67
heart disease, 43, 52, 58, 60, 104, 109
heavy metals, 45, 99, 107, 111. *See also* lead
Heidi (patient), 168–69
herbs
  Ayurveda and, 95, 97, 180, 184, 186, 198–99, 200
  infertility and, 156
  principles of integrative medicine and, 14
  spirituality and, 216, 217

supplements and, 94–98, 99
TCM and, 161, 169, 170, 174, 175, 176–77
See also specific herb
Heschel, Abraham Joshua, 214, 218
Hibbeln, Joseph, 72
homeopathy, 181
hormone replacement therapy, 66
hormones
  acupuncture and, 173
  Ayurveda and, 187, 189
  blood levels of, 37
  difficulty with conception and, 151, 152–53
  environmental impact on, 104
  exercise and, 44
  fertility problems and, 40, 44, 49
  function of, 124
  herbs and, 187, 189
  mind-body connection and, 123
  and multiple hormonal feedback loops, 124
  nutrition and, 76
  TCM and, 162, 173
  See also specific hormone
household products: environment and, 104, 105
hyperprolactinemia, 40
hypnosis/hypnotherapy, 11, 24, 49, 121–22, 127, 128, 139
hypothalamus
  acupuncture and, 172, 173
  Ayurveda and, 188
  environment and, 105
  fertility problems and, 42, 44
  herbs and, 99
  hypnosis and, 139
  lifestyle and, 42, 44
  mind-body connection and, 124, 125, 126, 139
  physiology of stress and, 124, 126
  reproductive physiology and, 29, 30

synergism and, 105
hysterosalpingogram, 154

ICSI (intracytoplasmic sperm injection), 13, 151
imagery. *See* visualization
imaging studies, 40
immune system, 14, 52, 92, 95, 105, 106–7, 113, 120, 133, 149, 188
immunizations, 18, 19, 21
India, Maizes' visit to, 181
infections, 40, 47, 151–52, 153–54
infertility
  complexity of, 159
  definition of, 214
  as God's punishment, 214
  spirituality and, 214
  See also specific topic
inflammation, 52, 58, 60–61, 64, 92, 154. *See also* anti-inflammatories; anti-inflammatory (Mediterranean) diet
insecticides. *See* pesticides/insecticides
Institute for Agriculture and Trade Policy, 106
Institute of Medicine, 91
insulin, 38, 39, 40, 42, 58–59, 64, 70, 95, 97, 125, 153
insulin-like growth factor-1 (IGF-1), 69, 125
integrative medicine
  benefits of, 3
  body's natural ability to heal and, 8
  challenges of fertility and, 2
  characteristics of, 2–3
  as commitment to care for whole person, 7, 8
  definition of, 7–8
  influence of TCM on, 162
  principles of, 2, 12–15, 221–22
  secondary infertility story and, 10–12

integrative medicine (*cont.*)
  as synthesis of conventional
    and alternative medicines,
    3, 7, 9–10
  as therapeutic partnership,
    8–9
  treatment options available in,
    23–25
interfallopian transfer, 215
intrauterine insemination (IUI),
  155
invasive technologies, 13–14
iodine, 21, 72, 85, 86, 88–89
IQ, 46, 72, 108, 223
iron, 18, 21, 24, 53, 72, 85, 86,
  90, 93, 101
IVF (in vitro fertilization)
  acupuncture and, 156, 158,
    172–74
  age and, 5, 156, 157
  Ayurveda and, 194, 200
  birth defects and, 155–56,
    157
  conventional medicine and,
    151, 152, 155–58
  difficulty with conception
    and, 151, 152
  fertility problems and, 40, 43,
    44, 45, 47
  how many times to attempt,
    157–58
  important decisions about,
    156–58
  infertility and, 155–56
  lifestyle and, 43, 44, 45, 47,
    222
  mind-body connection and,
    139
  miscarriages and, 157
  nutrition/diet and, 158, 222
  principles of integrative
    medicine and, 13, 222
  risks of, 155
  spirituality/religion and,
    202–4, 215
  stress and, 158
  success rate for, 157–58
  supplements and, 93

TCM and, 172–74, 176
treatment options and, 24

Jackson, Lisa, 111
Joanne (patient), 176
Joe (patient), 168–69
Jonathan (patient), 108
journaling, 18, 23, 30, 127, 134,
  138–39, 145, 189
Judaism, 215–17
Julie (patient), 173–74

Kabat-Zinn, Jon, 78
Kapha, 181–83, 186, 187, 189,
  198, 199
karma, 199–200
Kessler, David, 68
kidneys, 99, 116, 163, 165,
  166–67, 168, 170, 171,
  174, 176, 177, 179

L-arginine, 93, 100
labels
  on food, 65–66, 68, 82–83
  on personal care products, 112
  on supplements, 87–88, 101
laboratory work, basic, 149–50
Lad, Vasant, 180
LaRoche, Loretta, 134
Laura (patient), 174–76
lead, 19, 22, 77, 91, 105, 111,
  116
Lee, Ta-Ya, 164, 168, 169–70,
  175
Leila (patient), 135
letrozole, 121
LH (luteinizing hormone)
  Ayurveda and, 188
  fertility problems and, 39, 40,
    41, 44, 48
  herbs and, 95
  infertility and, 154, 155
  lifestyle and, 44, 48
  male fertility and, 41
  mind-body connection and,
    124, 125
  ovulation predictor kits and,
    37

reproductive physiology and,
  30, 31, 37
lifestyle
  Ayurveda and, 181, 183, 184
  conventional medicine and,
    148, 151, 156
  definition of integrative
    medicine and, 7
  difficulty with conception
    and, 151
  environment and, 105
  fertility problems and, 41–49
  and fertility treatment as all-
    consuming, 24–25
  genetics and, 223
  importance of, 222–23
  infertility and, 156
  initial assessment and, 15–16
  integrative medicine
    therapeutic relationship
    and, 9
  IVF and, 222
  mind-body connection and,
    133
  motivation for changes in,
    51–52
  self-assessment test and, 22
  TCM and, 166, 167
  See also alcohol; exercise;
    obesity; sleep; smoking;
    weight
liver, 165–66, 168, 176, 198
Low Dog, Tieraona, 94, 95, 96,
  97, 99, 100–101
low glycemic index, 39
Lupron, 172
luteal phase
  age and, 4
  Ayurveda and, 186, 193
  beginning and end of, 30, 31
  characteristics of, 31
  difficulty with conception
    and, 153
  fertility problems and, 38, 39,
    40, 43, 44, 48, 49
  herbs and, 95
  lifestyle and, 43, 44, 48
  shortened, 4

supplements and, 92–93
TCM and, 174, 177
timing of menstrual cycle
    and, 35
luteal phase defect (LPD),
    39–40, 44

Maca (herb), 97, 100
magnesium, 87, 93, 96
Maine: body burden study in,
    105
Maizes, Victoria
    goal of, 10, 16
    mind-body practices of,
        144–45
    patient's relationship with,
        8–9
    personal and professional
        background of, 4–5
    spirituality of, 204–5
    treatment plans of, 9–10
    visit to India of, 181
mantras, 131–32, 180, 184, 191
Margarelli, Paul, 173
Marie (patient), 150
marital/partnership relations,
    141–42, 179, 180, 185,
    206, 215
Markowitz (Ilana and Neil)
    family, 215–17
massage, 122, 161, 180, 184,
    198, 199
McGee, Leslie, 164, 167, 168,
    170, 172, 176
Mead, Margaret, 223
medications
    conventional medicine and,
        149, 152, 154
    over-the-counter, 18, 21
    prescription, 3, 11, 17, 21
    for stimulating ovulation, 40,
        152, 154, 172
medicine: purpose of, 161. *See
    also type of medicine*
meditation
    Ayurveda and, 184, 185,
        189–96, 199
    mind-body connection and,

127, 129, 131–32, 133,
    144
mindful, 168
Raisin Exercise, 78–79
secondary infertility story
    and, 11
self-assessment test and, 23
sleep and, 49
spirituality and, 204, 207
TCM and, 161, 168, 174–76
Mediterranean diet. *See*
    anti-inflammatory
    (Mediterranean) diet
melatonin, 48
Melissa (patient), 27–28
men
    acupuncture and, 177
    antioxidants and fertility in,
        68
    Ayurveda and, 188, 189, 194
    conventional medicine and,
        148, 149, 151, 153, 154
    dairy products and, 69
    environmental impact on,
        109, 114, 115, 151
    fertility problems and, 41, 42,
        45, 46, 47, 151, 154
    genetic issues and, 41
    lifestyle of, 42, 45, 46, 47, 151
    medications and, 149
    mind-body connection and,
        125, 142
    nutrition of, 68, 69, 76, 151
    reproductive physiology and,
        41
    stress and, 125
    supplements and, 99–101,
        148
    TCM and, 177
    treatment for infertility in, 151
    weight of, 19, 42, 151
    See also marital/partnership
        relations; sperm
menopause, 45, 162, 172
menstruation/menstrual cycle
    acupuncture and, 171–72
    age and, 37
    average length of, 28

Ayurveda and, 181, 186, 187,
    188, 191, 193, 194
birth control pills and, 17,
    23–24, 27, 28
conventional medicine and,
    150, 152
difficulty with conception
    and, 152
fertility problems and, 39
follicular phase and, 30, 31
herbs and, 94–95, 97
hormonal surge during, 30
identification of most fertile
    time and, 34–37
initial assessments and, 17
knowing your own, 28–33
lifestyle and, 43, 47
luteal phase of, 30, 31, 35
midcycle spotting and, 37
mind-body connection and,
    120–21, 122, 125, 126
need for reacquaintance with,
    4
normal, regular, 29
nutrition and, 67
oral contraceptives and, 28
ovulation during, 30
reproductive physiology and,
    28–33, 49
self-assessment test and, 20,
    22
shortening of, 37
supplements and, 93
TCM and, 28, 162, 163, 166,
    167, 171–72, 175
timing of, 34–35
variation in, 28, 34
West fertility journey and, 195
mercury, 19, 22, 24, 72–76, 77,
    105, 107, 108, 117
metals. *See* heavy metals
metformin, 91–92
microwaving, 109, 110
mikveh ritual, 207, 215
milk, 24, 69–70, 77, 98, 113
milk thistle, 98, 99, 198
mind
    Ayurveda and, 179, 180, 200

mind (*cont.*)
  cleansing and preparing, 179, 180
  definition of integrative medicine and, 7
  principles of integrative medicine and, 2, 222
  self-assessment of, 222
  See also mind-body connection
mind-body connection
  acupuncture and, 122, 223
  Ayurveda and, 180–81, 185, 189, 193, 194, 197
  belief system and, 136, 137–38
  blame and, 142–45
  body scanning and, 127, 129, 132
  breath work and, 119–20, 127–33, 144, 145
  cognitive behavioral therapy and, 125–26, 134, 140–41
  cognitive restructuring and, 127, 134–38
  conventional medicine and, 148
  environment and, 137, 143
  examples of mind-body connection and, 119–20
  exercise and, 122, 134, 138
  hypnosis and, 121–22, 127, 128, 139
  innate healing response of body and, 120
  integrative medicine and, 2, 3, 13, 222
  journaling and, 127, 134, 138–39, 145
  lifestyle and, 133
  marital/partnership relations and, 141–42
  meditation and, 127, 129, 131–32, 133, 144
  men and, 125, 142
  negativity and, 134, 135, 139
  personal practice/coping strategies for, 126–34, 142

placebos in clinical studies and, 120
  relaxation and, 127–34, 140–41, 144, 145
  self-assessment and, 23
  sleep and, 49
  spirituality and, 207
  stress and, 120, 121, 123–28, 134, 135, 138, 139, 140–41, 142, 143
  support groups and, 122, 127, 140–41
  Suzanne's story about, 120–23
  Three A's and, 144
  as tool for physicians, 9
  yoga and, 189, 197
mindfulness, 127, 138, 145, 168
Ming-Men area, 170, 179
miscarriages
  acupuncture and, 176
  age and, 4
  Ayurveda and, 186–87, 191, 192, 195
  diet and, 186–87
  difficulty with conception and, 153
  environmental impact on, 109
  fertility problems and, 39, 43, 154
  herbs and, 95, 96, 97
  infections and, 154
  initial assessment and, 17
  Integrative Medicine approach and, 2
  IVF and, 157
  obesity and, 43
  secondary infertility story and, 11
  self-assessment test and, 22
  spirituality and, 211–12, 213–14
  supplements and, 84, 89, 92
  TCM and, 168–69, 176
  West fertility journey and, 195
  yoga and, 191, 192
mittelschmerz, 34, 36
Monterey Bay Aquarium, 108

moral/ethical practices: Ayurveda and, 184–85
moxibustion: TCM and, 161, 170
MTHFR (methylenetetrahydrofolate reductase), 153
multiple births, 155, 157
multiple hormonal feedback loops, 124
multivitamins, 3, 18, 21, 24, 63, 68–69, 81–82, 83–87, 90, 101, 148, 149
mythology, 219–20

N-acetyl cysteine, 93–94
Naiman, Rubin, 25
Naparstek, Belleruth, 132
National Health and Nutrition Examination Survey (NHANES), 71–72, 81, 90
National Institute of Ayurveda, Yoga, Unani, Siddha, and Homeopathy (India), 181
National Institutes of Health (NIH), 72
National Products Association (NPA), 83
National Resources Defense Council, 72
National Sanitation Foundation (NSF), 83
National Sleep Foundation, 47
Natural Resources Defense Council (NRDC), 73
nature, 144, 202
negativity, 134, 135, 139
nervous system
  acupuncture and, 172
  autonomic, 124, 126, 129
  Ayurveda and, 191, 194, 197, 199
  environmental impact on, 106, 107–8, 114, 116
  mind-body connection and, 120, 123–24, 126, 128–29, 130, 133–34
  parasympathetic, 123–24, 128–29, 130, 194

spirituality and, 217
supplements and, 88
sympathetic, 120, 123–24, 128, 172, 194
neural tubes, 22, 38, 40, 84, 88, 149, 151, 153, 181
New York University Fertility Center, 127
Ney, Maggie, 94, 96–97, 98–99
Nurses' Health Study II (NHS), 43–44, 46, 47–48, 63–65, 67–68, 69, 71, 77, 83–84, 90, 108–9
nutrition
    alcohol and, 54, 63, 77–78
    anti-inflammatory diet and, 52–63, 68
    antioxidants and, 68–69
    and basic nutritional needs of average woman, 53–54
    beverages and, 54, 63, 70–71
    calories and, 53
    carbohydrates and, 53, 54, 58–59, 64, 65, 67–68, 70
    challenges to fertility and, 2
    coffee and, 54, 63, 70–71
    dairy products and, 64, 69–70
    definition of integrative medicine and, 8
    difficulty with conception and, 151
    fats and, 53, 54, 59–61, 63–64
    fertility and, 63–79
    fiber and, 53, 54, 61, 63, 76
    folic acid and, 88
    inflammation and, 52, 58, 60–61, 64
    men and, 68, 69, 76
    mindful eating and, 78–79
    omega-3 fatty acids and, 53, 54, 65, 71, 72, 76–77
    organic foods and, 53, 54, 62–63, 68–69, 70, 76–77
    overall principles for good health and, 52–63
    phytonutrients and, 53, 54, 61–62

principles of integrative medicine and, 2, 13
    protein and, 53, 54, 61, 65–67, 70
    research about, 63–78
    safe, clear foods and, 62–63
    seafood and, 53, 61, 71–76, 77
    self-assessment test and, 20–21
    sleep and, 66, 70
    as tool for physicians, 9
    trans fats and, 61, 63, 64–65
    vitamins/supplements and, 53, 61, 63, 68–69, 77, 81
    See also diet
nutritionists, 3, 24, 135

ob-gyns, 177
obesity, 2, 39, 42–43, 47, 52, 109, 151. See also weight
Oliver, Mary, 217–18
omega-3 fatty acids
    basic nutritional needs of average woman and, 53
    environment and, 103
    herbs and, 97
    importance of, 71
    initial assessment and, 18
    nutrition and, 53, 54, 65, 71, 72, 76–77
    as polyunsaturated fats, 60–61
    sources of, 71, 72, 76–77
    as supplement, 85, 86, 89–90, 100, 101
    treatment options and, 24
    See also fish oil
omega-6 fatty acids, 53, 60–61, 65, 89
omega-9 fatty acids, 89
1-methyl-folate, 153
organic food, 22, 53, 54, 62–63, 68–69, 70, 76–77, 98, 99, 107, 108, 110, 112, 186
organophosphates, 19
ovarian cancer, 155
ovarian cysts, 38
ovarian reserve, 151, 153

ovaries
    acupuncture and, 172
    Ayurveda and, 191
    environmental impact on, 105
    fertility problems and, 40–41, 42, 44
    infertility and, 154
    lifestyle and, 42, 44
    mind-body connection and, 124, 125, 126
    reproductive physiology and, 28
    TCM and, 164, 166, 172
    transposition of, 159
    See also egg(s); ovulation
overdiagnosis, 13
overtreatment, 13
ovulation
    conventional medicine and, 148, 151, 152, 153, 154
    diet and, 171
    difficulty with conception and, 151, 152, 153
    fertility problems and, 38, 40–41, 42
    identification of most fertile time and, 34
    importance of being acquainted with body and, 23
    medications for inducing, 40, 152, 154, 172
    mind-body connection and, 124, 125, 126
    obesity and, 42
    reproductive physiology and, 30, 34–35, 36
    TCM and, 171, 175
    See also ovulation predictor kit
ovulation predictor kit, 30, 34, 37, 148, 152

packaging: environment and, 109–10
PAH (polycyclic aromatic hydrocarbons), 113

panchakarma. *See* Ayurveda: detoxification and
pap smears, 40
partridge berry, 96–97
Patanjali, 191
Patel, Premal, 185, 189, 194
patients
  doctor's relationship with, 8–9, 12, 24, 202, 221
  history of, 15–20
  initial assessments of, 15–20
  self-assessment of, 20–23, 222
  as telling story in own words, 16–17
Patton, Sharayle, 117
Paulus, Wolfgang, 173
PBDEs (brominated flame retardants), 105, 116–17
PCBs, 19, 22, 77, 90, 108
PCOS (polycystic ovarian syndrome)
  age for having a baby and, 4
  Ayurveda and, 181, 186
  conventional medicine and, 150, 153
  fertility problems and, 27, 38–39, 40, 42, 49, 153
  herbs and, 97
  initial assessment and, 17, 19
  mind-body connection and, 121
  nutrition and, 59, 68, 70
  obesity and, 42
  ovulation predictor kits and, 37
  self-assessment test and, 22
  supplements and, 91–92, 93
  symptoms of, 38–39
  TCM and, 177
pediatric cancer, 84
pelvic area: warming of, 169–70
perchlorate, 89, 111
Perron, Joanne, 106, 108
Persephone (mythological goddess), 219
personal care products, 22, 24, 105, 112–13, 149
personal practice/coping

strategies, 126–34, 141. *See also specific practice*
pesticides/insecticides, 22, 62, 65, 99, 107, 110, 114–15
pharmaceuticals, 9, 10. *See also* medications
Pharmacopeia, U.S., 94
Pharmacopeial Convention, U.S. (USP), 83
Phelps-Sandall, Barbi, 153, 154
phthalates, 104, 105, 109, 110, 111, 113, 114
physical activity. *See* exercise
physicians
  discussions about likelihood of conception and, 149–50
  importance of listening by, 16, 17
  initial assessment by, 15–20
  open-mindedness of, 222–23
  patient's relationship with, 8–9, 12, 24, 202, 221
  role in integrative medicine of, 8–9
  spirituality and, 202
  as walking their talk, 12, 15, 222–23
physiology, reproductive
  age and, 35, 37–38
  identification of most fertile time and, 34–37
  knowing your menstrual cycle and, 28–33
  timing of menstrual cycle and, 34–35
phytoestrogens, 66, 67
phytonutrients, 53, 54, 61–62
Pitta, 181–83, 185, 186, 187, 188, 199
pituitary gland
  acupuncture and, 172, 173
  Ayurveda and, 188
  difficulty with conception and, 152
  environmental impact on, 105
  fertility problems and, 38, 39, 41, 42, 44

herbs and, 99
lifestyle and, 42, 44
male fertility and, 41
mind-body connection and, 124, 125
reproductive physiology and, 28, 30
placenta, 31, 107
plastics: environment and, 105, 109, 110, 111
postpartum depression, 60, 71, 89
potassium, 87, 97
prakruti. *See* balance: Ayurveda and
pranayama (breathing exercises), 130, 131, 190, 197–98
prayer, 2, 128, 131–32, 189, 195, 202, 203, 204, 205, 213–14, 217–18, 223
"Praying" (Oliver poem), 217–18
preeclampsia, 43, 91, 157
premature birth, 2, 45–46, 155, 157
President's Cancer Panel, 62
preterm labor, 11, 89, 148
prevention, health, 12, 15
probiotics, 92, 99
progesterone
  dairy products and, 69
  difficulty with conception and, 152–53
  fertility problems and, 39, 40
  herbs and, 95, 97
  mind-body connection and, 124, 126
  reproductive physiology and, 31
  secondary infertility story and, 11
  supplements and, 93
  TCM and, 177
progressive muscle relaxation, 49, 133
prolactin, 38, 47, 48, 69, 95, 97, 152–53, 173, 188
prostate cancer, 76, 109

protein, 21, 53, 54, 61, 63, 65–67, 70, 108–9, 170
Provera, 121, 122

qi, 163, 165–67, 168, 170, 171, 176, 177, 179, 180
qi gong, 161, 168

Rachel (biblical woman), 221
Rachel's Network, 104
radiation therapy, 159
radon, 111
Raisin Exercise, 78–79
reactive oxygen species (ROS), 83
red clover flower, 96
red raspberry leaf, 96
relaxation
    acupuncture and, 172, 173
    mind-body connection and, 127–34, 140–41, 144, 145
    need for culture of, 133
    spirituality and, 217–18
    TCM and, 167, 172, 173
religion, 212–14, 215–17
Remen, Rachel Naomi, 201–2
reproductive technology
    activism and, 223
    age and, 3–4, 223
    making decisions about, 222
    religion and, 215
    See also assisted reproduction; specific technology
retreats: mind-body connection and, 144–45
rituals. See ceremonies/rituals
Rubenstein, David, 216

salt, 21, 88–89
saunas, 98
saw palmetto, 97
schisandra, 99
science: principles of integrative medicine and, 12, 13, 14–15
seafood
    basic nutritional needs of average woman and, 53

environment and, 107–8, 117
FDA-recommended amount of, 72
fertility and, 71–76
mercury in, 72–76, 107–8, 117
nutrition and, 53, 61, 71–76, 77
self-assessment test and, 21, 22
treatment options and, 24
See also omega-3 fatty acids; sushi
secondary infertility, Garrison's, 10–12
Seeger, Susan, 136–37
Self-Assessment Test, 20–23, 222
self-care, 9, 133, 173, 179
self-image, 141
Sertoli cells, 41
Sethi, Tanmeet, 185, 188, 194, 199
sexual activity, 34, 166–67
sexual dysfunction, 140. See also erectile dysfunction
sexually transmitted diseases (STDs), 40
Seychelles Islands: fish study in, 72
Sgarlata, Carl, 147–48, 153, 154–55, 156, 158, 159
Shah, Falguni, 179–80
shakuyaku-kanzo-to (herb), 97
Shambhala Mountain Center (Colorado), 189
shampoos, 22, 24
shatavari (herb), 95–96, 97, 180, 187–88
SHBG (sex hormone-binding globulin), 39, 42, 47, 58–59, 69
Shere-Wolfe, Kalpana, 202–4, 217
Shere-Wolfe, Kiran, 204
Silverman, Howard, 207–8, 209
skin cancer, 91
sleep
    coffee/caffeine and, 70

environmental impact on, 105–6
fertility problems and, 47–49
herbs and, 98
"let go" into, 49
mind-body connection and, 141
Naiman's views about, 25
nutrition and, 66, 70
principles of integrative medicine and, 13
self-assessment test and, 22
suggestions for getting a good night's, 48–49
TCM and, 164, 166
smoking, 19, 22, 45–46, 49, 51, 148, 151
soda/soft drinks, 54, 71, 175
solvents, 19, 22
sonohystogram, 154
soy regimen, 66–67
Sparrowe, Linda, 189–90, 192, 197
sperm
    Ayurveda and, 188
    conventional medicine and, 148, 149
    count of, 41, 47, 99, 109, 114, 115, 153, 177, 188
    difficulty with conception and, 151, 153
    environmental impact on, 109, 114, 115
    fertility problems and, 41, 45
    herbs and, 188
    infertility and, 155
    lifestyle and, 47
    medications affecting, 149
    physiology of stress and, 125
    quality of, 177, 188
    reproductive physiology and, 35
    smoking and, 45
    supplements and, 99–100, 148
    survival time of, 35
    TCM and, 177
    See also ICSI

spirit/spirituality
  Ayurveda and, 179, 180–81, 200
  ceremonies/rituals and, 205–12, 219
  cleansing and preparing the, 179
  connected feelings and, 209, 210–11
  definition of integrative medicine and, 7
  definition of, 201–2
  fertility and, 215–17
  importance of, 201
  infertility and, 214
  initial assessment and, 19–20
  marital/partnership relations and, 206
  meditation and, 204, 207
  mind-body connection and, 144, 207
  mystery of birth and, 205, 222
  mythology and, 219–20
  nature and, 202
  physician-patient relationship and, 202
  prayer and, 202, 203, 204, 205, 213–14, 217–18
  principles of integrative medicine and, 2
  relaxation and, 217–18
  religion and, 212–14, 215–17
  self-assessment test and, 23, 222
  sense of gratitude and, 218
spleen, 166, 168, 176
Standard American Diet (SAD), 60, 171
stillbirth, 89, 157
stinging nettle, 96, 99
strawberries, 107
stress
  acupuncture and, 172, 173
  Ayurveda and, 184, 185, 186, 188
  becoming an activist and, 223
  challenges to fertility and, 2

conventional medicine and, 148, 158
definition of integrative medicine and, 8
environment and, 105, 106, 113
excessive, 40
exercise and, 44
fertility problems and, 38, 40, 44
herbs and, 95, 98, 101, 188
hormone-disrupting, 2
inflammation and, 52
initial assessment and, 19
IVF and, 158
men and, 125
mind-body connection and, 120, 121, 123–28, 134, 135, 138, 139, 142, 143
multiple small, 126
oxidative, 38, 83, 99, 100, 113
physiology of, 123–26
principles of integrative medicine and, 2, 15, 222
role in enhancing fertility of, 140–41
self-assessment test and, 23
self-care and, 9
sperm count and, 99
supplements and, 83, 99, 100
TCM and, 163, 167–68, 172, 173, 174, 175, 179
yoga and, 190
stress-induced anovulation (SIA), 125
sudden infant death syndrome, 46
supplements
  conventional medicine and, 148, 149
  detoxification and, 98–99
  fertility problems and, 40
  initial assessment and, 18
  labels on, 87–88, 101
  lifestyle and, 28
  for men, 99–101, 148
  nutrition and, 53, 61, 63, 68–69, 77, 81

prevalence of use of, 81–82
principles of integrative medicine and, 2, 13
regulation of, 82–83
secondary infertility story and, 11
selection of, 101
self-assessment test and, 21
sources of information about, 21
See also vitamins; specific supplement
support groups, 122, 127, 140–41, 222
surgery, 9, 22
surrogate motherhood, 215, 221, 222
Susan (patient), 23–24
sushi, 24, 72–75, 117
Suzanne (patient), 120–23, 128
synergism, 105
synthetic musks, 113

tai chi, 120, 127, 129
tea, 49, 54, 63, 93, 171
teflon, 105, 110
temperature. See Basal Body Temperature (BBT)
Temple Stay, 110
testicles, 41, 47, 104, 124, 125, 151
testosterone, 39, 41, 42, 47, 59, 69, 97, 109, 124, 125, 149
tests/testing
  basic, 149–50
  risks of diagnostic, 14
  See also type of test
tetracycline, 149
The Three A's, 144
three vital substances
  TCM and, 163, 165–66
  See also specific substance
thyroid
  Ayurveda and, 188
  conventional medicine and, 149, 150
  difficulty with conception and, 153

environmental impact on, 104, 108
fertility problems and, 38, 40
initial assessment and, 19
iodine and, 88, 89
mind-body connection and, 124, 125, 126
nutrition and, 68
reproductive physiology and, 28
self-assessment test and, 21
supplements and, 88, 89
toxins: testing for, 117
Trachelospermum (herb), 189
Traditional Chinese Medicine (TCM)
    acupuncture and, 161, 169, 171–76, 177
    assessment and, 223
    balance and, 161–62, 171–76, 178
    blood in, 163, 165–67, 176
    core beliefs of, 163
    diet/food and, 161, 166, 167, 170–71, 179
    energy and, 162, 165, 166–67, 168, 169, 170, 171, 174, 176, 177
    enhancement of fertility with, 177–78
    essence in, 163–64, 165–67, 170, 171, 176
    fertility and, 40, 210, 216
    gardening metaphor and, 161–62
    goal of, 162
    herbs and, 97, 161, 169, 170, 174, 175, 176–77
    infertility and, 156, 162–63, 165
    IVF and, 172–74, 176
    meditation and, 161, 168, 174–76
    men and, 177
    menstruation and, 28, 162, 163, 166, 167, 171–72, 175
    miscarriages and, 168–69, 176
    as option for treatment plan, 9
    in practice, 168–78
    preparation for pregnancy and, 2
    qi and, 163, 165–67, 168, 170, 171, 176, 177, 179
    relaxation and, 167, 172, 173
    spirituality and, 210, 216
    stress and, 163, 167–68, 172, 173, 174, 175, 179
    synthesis of integrative medicine and, 3, 162
    theory of, 163–67
    three vital substances and, 163, 165–67
    Western medicine compared with, 161, 163–64
    yin and yang and, 163, 164, 166, 167, 171, 172, 177, 178
trans fats, 61, 63, 64–65
treatments
    options available for, 9–10, 23–25
    physician-patient relationship and selection of, 23–24
    principles of integrative medicine and, 13
    risks and side effects of, 13
triglycerides, 39
triplets, 157
TSH (thyroid-stimulating hormone), 150
tui na (massage), 161
turmeric, 99, 187, 188–89
Turner's syndrome, 41
twins, 88, 157

ultrasound, 37, 40, 151, 152, 154
University of Pune (India), 187–88
ureaplasma, 154
uterus, 39, 40, 41, 154, 172

vagina, 30, 35
vaginal cancer, 104
vegans, 86, 91, 195
vegetarians, 67, 170
Vietnam War, 82
visualization, 28, 49, 119, 127, 136–37, 202, 203, 207
vitamin A, 86, 87–88, 96
vitamin B, 87, 93
vitamin B$_{12}$, 87, 91–92, 93
vitamin C, 11, 86, 87, 91, 92–93, 99, 100
vitamin D, 18, 21, 24, 77, 86, 91, 96, 97, 100, 101, 149
vitamin E, 87, 99, 100
vitamins, 2, 53, 68–69, 77. *See also* multivitamins; supplements; *specific vitamin*
Vitex agnus-castus. See chasteberry
vitrification technique, 158
vulva, 35, 37

walking, 44, 138, 145
Wallinga, David, 106, 113, 115
warming of pelvic area, 169–70
water, 54, 63, 98, 110–12, 116
water bottles, 98, 105, 109, 111
weight
    Ayurveda and, 186
    birth, 46, 113, 114, 157
    challenges to fertility and, 2
    conventional medicine and, 148, 150, 157
    detoxification and, 98
    fertility problems and, 2, 39, 43, 45, 46, 47, 49
    initial assessment and, 18–19
    lifestyle and, 45, 46, 47
    nutrition and, 52
    principles of integrative medicine and, 15, 222
    self-assessment test and, 22, 23
    See also obesity
Weil, Andrew, 4, 130, 198
West, De, 192–96, 197
Westphal, Lynn, 93
whole foods. *See* organic food

Willett, Walter, 63
World Health Organization, 89, 115
worry, 59, 119, 148, 150, 166, 168

X chromosome, 41
X-rays, 19, 22

Yang, Jingduan, 165, 166–67, 168, 174
yin and yang, 163, 164, 166, 167, 171, 172, 177, 178, 180

yoga
Ayurveda and, 180, 184–85, 189–96, 197–98, 199
breath work and, 181, 189, 190, 191, 192, 194, 196, 197–98
mind-body connection and, 120, 127, 129, 130, 144, 145
philosophy of, 194
pointers about, 190–92, 196
poses in, 189–94, 195, 197, 217
rigorous, 192, 196

secondary infertility story and, 11
self-assessment test and, 23
spirituality and, 204, 210, 216, 217
stress and, 190
TCM and, 174–76
West fertility journey and, 194–96
yogurt, 70, 92

Zhang, Qingcai, 161
zinc, 87, 93, 97, 99–100

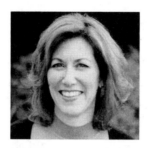

About the Author

Dr. Victoria Maizes is Executive Director of the Arizona Center for Integrative Medicine and Professor of Medicine, Family and Community Medicine, and Public Health at the University of Arizona.

Chosen by Dr. Andrew Weil to lead the Arizona Center for Integrative Medicine in 2000, Dr. Maizes is internationally recognized as a leader in integrative medicine. She stewarded the growth of the Center for Integrative Medicine, which now educates 250 fellows and residents annually. She helped develop the Center's curriculum in integrative medicine and pioneered multiple educational innovations, including Integrative Family Medicine and Integrative Medicine in Residency, two national models for educating primary-care physicians.

A graduate of Barnard College, Dr. Maizes received her MD from the University of California, San Francisco, and completed her residency in Family Medicine at the University of Missouri, Columbia, and her Fellowship in Integrative Medicine at the University of Arizona.

Dr. Maizes lectures worldwide to academic and community audiences on integrative medicine, women's health, fertility, healthy aging, nutrition, and cancer. She was co-editor of the Oxford University Press textbook *Integrative Women's Health,* and in 2009 she was named one of the world's 25 Intelligent Optimists by *ODE Magazine.* A mother of three, she lives in Tucson, Arizona, with her family.